Judas Dentistry

How Dentists Scorn Science, Break the Hippocratic Oath, and Wreck Their Patients' Minds and Bodies

Robert Yoho, MD

Inverness Press

Contents

Part Two

Judas Dentists Live Inside the Rockefeller Medicine Matrix

Praise and reader comments

About Dr. Yoho's writing.

✪ So many academics have quietly thumbed their noses at medical doctors for years, hence why none of my PhD friends call themselves doctors. —GL

✪ I want to thank you for writing this book. I am a victim of numerous experiences with dentists and the specialists involved in dentistry. I have suffered so much physically and mentally that I am amazed I am still here. —YT

✪ I had part of a dentist-damaged tooth broke off two days ago. I haven't gone to dentists in years because of the damage they do and the cost. A sealer or resin filling would take care of the tooth, but I could not find a dentist who would simply do that. It is a crime that Weston Price's work has not been the rule for dentistry from his time. He discovered that proper eating yields healthy, solid bones and teeth. Thanks for getting the word out. —JR

✪ I used to get so many fillings—it's a miracle my teeth are still in my mouth. About ten years ago, I realized I was eating horribly and causing myself chronic disease. I learned about the microbiome and how important good bacteria are to the human body, and I completely changed my diet. My tooth decay stopped after cutting out refined grains, sugar, processed meat, food additives, and other processed foods like vegetable oils. I no longer have receding gums. I also increased my veggies, legumes, and other nutrient-packed foods. I now use clay-based toothpaste that tastes terrible but helps mineralize the teeth. I floss at least once a day. I have decent gaps that food gets stuck in. I doubt I even need the toothpaste now. I eat a diet that supports healthy bacteria living in my mouth, and my body no longer has to rob calcium from my teeth and bones to buffer itself from being overly acidic. —KL

✪ With everything going on, it sure seems like they have been trying to poison us for many decades. Your body will eliminate some of this, but we cannot know what might remain. Thanks for another "health" area I can no longer trust. —FD

✪ Fantastic post, Dr. Yoho. I'm 100% with you on dental and body care. The baking soda can sting for the first few days as your body acclimates. One suggestion: I've not done the in-depth research, but finding another brand than Arm & Hammer, such as Bob's Red Mill, might be a better practice. It is not cheap and doesn't come in 13-pound bags, but I'm guessing it's processed with fewer impurities. In a similar vein, showering every day in chlorinated water is another habit that should be stopped. Getting a filter on the shower head is a simple solution. —SD

✪ I changed to a biological dentist about ten years ago. I removed all amalgams and root canals. I'm so thankful I have this resource where I live. I buy all personal care products at the local health food store and get a couple of prescriptions from a local compounding pharmacy. When I see pharmacies like CVS and Walgreens, I see McDonald's medicine. Junk! —MC

✪ Yup. I had all the amalgams removed from my mouth about 14 years ago by my ex, the holistic dentist. I immediately felt better, slept better, had less anxiety, and I could drink hot or cold liquids without pain. You're spot on! —CF

✪ A few months ago, I had the best dental cleaning in my life. The hygienist had already recommended a hydroflosser and Dental Herb oil for gum inflammation, so I started using a Waterpik. Instead of using a lot of the oil ($40 per bottle), I started brushing with baking soda and then using hydrogen peroxide in the Waterpik water. I had the least amount of plaque ever, especially in my lower front teeth, which was always torture to remove. —AS

✪ Good on you, Dr. Yoho. I was going to say "good luck" but realized that luck would have very little to do with it. I'm your age. I had quite a few amalgams and used to suffer from migraines. Funnily enough, not being a celeb follower and a rebel all my life, when I heard that Princess Diana had hers removed, I decided to have mine removed as well. It was done with the proper protection, too. It took some 6-7 months for the migraines to vanish. —WT

✪ Thank you, Robert, for this excellent summary. The door to our health opens with our mouth. Bugs, bugs everywhere... I wonder how you start with a good colonization. Gums need L. acidophilus so much; I wonder why Covid is connected with the same type of missing bacteria. The same one we get at birth, which is now gone? —EJ

✪ SMART is a global health initiative to protect dental patients, dental employees, and the global environment from the harmful effects of mercury that is generated during the removal of dental amalgam fillings, which contain roughly 50% elemental mercury. https://thesmartchoice.com/ —MR

✪ Dentistry is the subject that started my questioning of medicine and drugs 12 years ago. Covid was the nail in the coffin of my trust. I'm not even sure my functional medicine doctor is correct on much now, either. I've dropped mucho money on him. I'm backing off now as I'm learning to treat myself. I've always thought dentists were highly paid butchers. —RI

✪ I vacuum up every word, phrase, and sentence from every post of yours, Dr. Yoho, and am about to pull the trigger on buying all of your books. I've never seen such a thorough warning list of all the dangers of "modern healthcare." Thank you, kind sir, for this thoughtful and well-researched essay #275, "Almost Everything Scares Me These Days." Caveat Emptor! - Let the buyer beware! — NV

✪ I am 81 and a retired Special Forces officer. I run a small shooting school with unarmed defensive tactics near Durango, CO. I was recently attracted to the carnivore world, and an awful lot has come my way through your site. When the government came out against hydroxychloroquine, I knew something was off. I and my peers had been issued Chloroquine primaquine for our time in the tropics, and the only problem was a few involuntary bowel movements. We took it once a week and safely. I remain unvaxxed! My research led me to Quercetin as a substitute for hydroxychloroquine as an ionophore, Dr. Z, and so on. God bless you and keep on pushing. —RS

✪ I got a sunlight lamp in 1996 after struggling through every winter. It was a big box that cost $400, but it worked within a week, and hubby wondered who this new woman was. My seasonal affective disorder has dissipated, mostly because I'm outdoors often in the winter. My vitamin D is high, and I live a happier, more fulfilled life. These lights can be very effective for many. —LS

✪ Wow. Excellent article & info. I worked 15 years in healthcare, and none of it ever sat right with me... It always felt more like slow death care. I just couldn't put it all together and was busy raising two boys while working—a shameful situation. I'll never go back. Thank you! I am ordering your books now!!!! —YR

✪ Dr. Yoho, thank you!! This is one of the most essential postings on Substack. It is a comprehensive examination of our Predatory Sick Care System. Hats off! Kudos! You have done your homework. Though I have been aware of most contained here, there are some new critical additions to my knowledge base. It is powerful. Thank you again for your masterpiece! Keep cranking! Great job on that speed ascent on El Cap, too. Strong, brother!! —KR

✪ Dr. Yoho always offers a Substack filled with helpful information I'm not coming across elsewhere, at least not in breadth.—SH.

✪ First of all, I LOVE the climbing shot!! [Reproduced in Chapter 14 of *Judas Dentistry*.] Tim and I were mere novices compared to you. And drill, fill, and bill—I'm sure my teenage mouth was used for this racketeering nonsense. I'm still on the fence about widening and drilling out healthy remaining tooth structure and weakening what is left to change the filling—thinking on this. —UJ

✪ Your books have taught me so much this last year. Thank you 🙏. —TP

✪ Brother. Thank you. We have become an increasingly paranoid world where we think science and chemicals can save us. They cannot. We are told day after day how and where to live. We are earth's creatures. I am not afraid of the sun. At 66, I still dig in the earth with my hands, walk on the beach, and feel the grass on my bare feet. And yes. I step in dog poo. It washes off. I don't like snow, but I will endure it. —RT

✪ Dr. Y, thank you for your honesty and excellent writing skills. I recently attended a reunion lunch with several ER nurse friends. It's sad to report most took the Covid jab. DFL and DFR (don't freaking listen and don't freaking read) —SY

✪ Thank you! Fantastic information, as usual! I will speculate that any amelioration of allergies would come from cleaning up the gut and helping immune functioning. We will try it at some point. We have spent tens of thousands of dollars in functional medicine trying to get my son to be less allergic (he has Eosinophilic Esophagitis.). He is very disciplined, in his early twenties, and manages without pharmaceuticals via an elimination diet and many supplements. This means he can safely eat only about 25 to 30 foods. Never eats at restaurants. He has environmental and chemical allergies as well. EoE was unheard of 40 years ago. It has exploded along the timeline of the increase in childhood vaccine uptake. LDA and LDI (low dose allergen) therapy are suppressed treatments for allergies but, unfortunately, did not work for my son. They are available through independent practicing integrative medicine MDs. —LR

✪ Thank you, thank you, Dr. Yoho. I will try chlorine dioxide for my high mercury and encourage friends with Lyme to try it, too.......and for many other things. When assembling my supplies, I will do multiples for Christmas gifts and your excellent article. Great article!!!!!!! 10 Stars. It was so complete, and you made it so easy. —BT

✪ This is a great dental information article. Welcome to the club of doctors who help patients obtain and maintain health and vitality. I would second all the information in this newsletter. Dentists are deadly to most of their patients. They are one of the only medical professionals who leave dead body parts in their patients' bodies. I, too, was trained by Dr. Huggins on cavitation surgeries and tried to practice holistically. I wrote a dental health care book in 2018 that attempted to give people a summary of what to do to take care of themselves without a lot of dental intrusions. It was called Holistic Dental Care. I will check out the websites you listed. I have started a Substack newsletter for like-minded health practitioners and would love your input. —Blessings, Rev. Dr. Stephen A. Lawrence.

✪ Thank you for this profoundly impactful information, Dr. Yoho. I will be sure to read your other articles regarding criminal conventional dentistry and share this far and wide. —HS

✪ Horrible is putting it mildly. Although, given all the fraudulent theories we're encouraged to subscribe to by allopathic medicine, I guess it's hardly surprising. Thanks again for your tireless efforts, Dr. Yoho. And, from the bottom of a single mother's heart, double thanks for keeping your Substack free. —VT

✪ I am deeply moved by the sled dog post. Your erudition strikes me. Your references to classical literature are so nourishing I feel your love coming through. I also admire and respect your vulnerability. The post is like a loving father saying don't do what I did. Pause, rest, reflect, recharge. —KR

✪ I did not realize bad teeth could be so harmful to health. Incidentally, I have never been to a dentist in 40 years, not since my last compulsory primary school visit. I have never had any real health issues since that time. I am now more resolved to continue my dentist-free life. On the fluoride: I think its use in drinking water may be a cause for older women's fragile bones; lifelong consumption of fluoride water could result in the bone destruction that is drilled (haha) into us. —OV

About the Cover

Judas was the Apostle who was given 30 pieces of silver to betray Jesus's identity to the people who had come to arrest him. Dentists are paid handsomely for using damaging treatments on those who trust them.

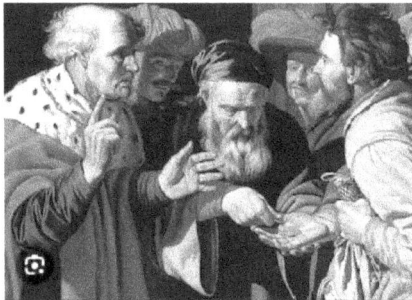

The Payment of Judas (mid-1600s), by Gerard Seghers.

Also by Dr. Yoho

A New Body in One Day (2004)

Butchered by "Healthcare" (2020)

Hormone Secrets (2021).

Cassandra's Memo (2023)

Twenty articles in medical journals, including;

The American Journal of Cosmetic Surgery   Vol. 20, No. 3, 2003   149

Modified Propofol-Ketamine Cosmetic Surgery: Anesthesia Technique for Surgeon-Administered Anesthesia With Particular Reference to Liposuction

Robert Yoho, MD; Kevin Mullen, PA

Review   > Dermatol Surg. 2005 Jul;31(7 Pt 1):733-43; discussion 743.
doi: 10.1097/00042728-200507000-00001.

Review of the liposuction, abdominoplasty, and face-lift mortality and morbidity risk literature

Robert A Yoho [1], Jeremy J Romaine, Deborah O'Neil

Cosmetic surgery website: I retired in 2019, but DrYoho.com is still live. Author website: RobertYohoAuthor.com

Judas Dentistry

How Dentists Scorn Science, Break the Hippocratic
Oath, and Wreck Their Patients' Minds and Bodies

By Robert Yoho, MD (ret)
Editor: Elizabeth Cronin, JD

Editing credit: KEC

For information, contact RobertYohowriter@gmail.com

Robert Yoho

PO Box 50007

Pasadena, California, 91115

ISBN ebook: 978-1-7354857-9-9 $3.99

Free download here: https://dl.bookfunnel.com/5ercuvl94y

ISBN paperback: 979-8-9898176-0-3 $25.00

BISAC Subject Codes:

MED035000 MEDICAL / Health Care Delivery

HEA028000 HEALTH & FITNESS / Health Care Issues

BUS070170 BUSINESS & ECONOMICS / Industries / Healthcare

The stories here came from actual patients or doctors, who all gave permission. I changed some names and a few details to preserve their privacy.

$25.00

ISBN 979-8-9898176-0-3

52500>

9 798989 817603

Paperback.

978-1-7354857-9-9 Ebook

"Legal" Disclaimer

I have no conflicts of interest that I can identify. I am not soliciting business for myself —I retired from practice when I was 66 and resigned my medical license. I had a fantastic career as a cosmetic surgeon, and I was initially sad to end it. But I am happy that a small part of my life is left to write, research, and contribute.

I have no financial relationship with any doctor or institution, nor have I received funding from anyone. I do not own substantial healthcare stock. If there are any net profits from this book, I will donate them to a worthy cause.

These are my opinions based on decades of medical training, practice, and reading the literature. I make no guarantees about them; none of this book should be construed as assessment, diagnosis, treatment, or medical advice. Your licensed providers are the only ones who should advise you, but you must learn as much as possible and take your own counsel as well. I cannot recommend any specific doctor in this age of frivolous lawsuits. Remember that each has an individual license, and they, not I, are responsible for your treatment.

To my friends who turned disasters into lifetimes of service. Here is an Aurelius quote for each of you.

Becky Dutton, *Metals Goddess.*
"Bad luck borne nobly is good luck."

Robert Gammal *is the dentist who stepped out of the Matrix.*
"Nothing hinders you from doing what must be done."

J, my anonymous colleague, *walks with equanimity among psychopaths. You gave me a gift I can never repay.*
"With the god's wind beating on our backs, we pull harder on the oars and make no complaint."

How to Read This Book

This manuscript is only 44,000 words, and I recommend reading every bit. It is about your health, and you are worth the effort.

✪ I have a quirky habit of inserting loosely related stories into my writing as "Intermissions" or "Parting Shots" after some chapters. My themes are so brutal that you need occasional breaks.

✪ The references are available as links in the ebook, which you can access free HERE (https://dl.bookfunnel.com/5ercuvl94y). These links cannot be accessed from the print or PDF versions. To find the original, unedited posts and their audio on RobertYoho.Substack.com, focus your cellphone camera on the QR code at the start of the chapters. Or, from the ebook, click the "LINK" below this.

✪ I am not a nonprofit; I am a *no-profit*. I give what I make here to whoever I think will help our health and world freedom the most, and I send all net Amazon funds to my Amazon Ads contractor.

Freebies and more

Thank you!

✪ To access the references in my books as links, download the ebooks as my gifts. The only favor I ask in return is that you pass the download links to at least five people. HERE is how to download my viral hit, *Butchered by "Healthcare."* For *Hormone Secrets*, the link is HERE. Both of these are Amazon bestsellers. *Cassandra's Memo* is HERE, and a podcast about it is HERE.

✪ The audio version of the first half of *Butchered by "Health-care"* is published as a free podcast HERE and on YouTube. You can also listen to the first half of *Hormone Secrets* on YouTube HERE.

✪ Buy my books, and Amazon will prioritize your reviews. On Amazon: *Hormone Secrets* is HERE, and *Butchered by "Health-care"* is HERE. THIS is the secret link on Amazon for *Cassandra's Memo*, and it is also available at Barnes and Noble HERE.

Substack

This is not yet censored.

✪ It is now worth more dead than alive, so a predator may buy it and pull the plug. If that happens, I will make my content available elsewhere. To stay with me, be sure I have your email by subscribing to Surviving Healthcare at RobertYoho.Substack.com. I will send you updates. RobertYohoAuthor.com has more.

✪ To search my archives, go to RobertYoho.Substack.com and use the pulldown archive menu at the upper right and the search box.

✪ To discuss my posts, please reply in the comments rather than using email. Aggressive disagreements are welcome, but insincerity is not. If I suspect you of that, I will bounce you.

Podcasts

I have been a guest on hundreds. THIS one is about hormone supplementation. A hormone testimonial video is HERE. A podcast about healthcare corruption is HERE, and THIS is an introduction to *Butchered by "Healthcare."*

All my best,

Robert Yoho, MD
   Yoho.robert@gmail.com
   May 2024

Research Tips

For any reader.

✪ Although "link rot" destroys up to ten percent of the Internet's content yearly, virtually everything posted is still alive and well on the Wayback Internet Archive. Not even the Chinese or the global psychopaths have so far been able to hide from it. To find a hidden link, copy the bad URL (the original web address) and enter it at archive.org. Then, look for the backed-up copies and select the date you want to view. You can also save any page indefinitely for free on another of their pages.

Unfortunately, the Wayback may soon be vandalized or even destroyed. Learn more about this in Chapter 8, Fake Fact Checking of *Cassandra's Memo*.

✪ All information—of any kind—should be shared freely. Secrecy, especially by governments, enables crime. Blasting through certain paywalls is easy; https://www.removepaywall.com/ works as of this publication.

✪ Another option is Sci-hub, a "piracy" website in Russia that can get you many academic articles free if you copy the link into their browser. This is against US law, but some academics publicly thank them. Whether you pay for articles is a private matter between you, Sci-hub, the journal, and your maker. Rumors of Sci-hub's demise may be premature, but they are repeatedly changing their domain endings as they are seized. Try sci-hub.ru. More HERE.

Preface

I knew nothing about dentists until the last half of 2023. I was forced to study them when I realized they had crippled my health. You will see how my thinking evolved as I researched and interviewed experts.

When I was nine, I met my first "tooth doctor" during the "drill, fill, and bill" era. In those days, they were jamming mercury amalgams into every natural tooth pit and crevice they could find. Although I never had pain, our dentist always managed to convince my obsessive mother that my mouth was packed with cavities. By adulthood, I had 17 "silver fillings."

In mid-2023, after a decade of a left-handed tremor that seemed merely annoying, a neurologist diagnosed me with Parkinson's disease (PD). Mercury is the most common cause; my tests showed this, as well as lead, aluminum, chromium, and glyphosate. Few neurologists have a clue that pollutants such as these, paraquat, and Agent Orange cause PD, autism, Alzheimer's, multiple sclerosis, and amyotrophic lateral sclerosis. They dub these "syndromes" because the origins are supposedly unknown. Corporate medicine rarely looks for cures; instead, diseases are named, and the symptoms are treated long-term with profitable drugs.

To learn what to do, I studied aggressively. First, I had my mercury amalgams removed. More recently, I have been getting intravenous phosphatidylcholine followed by glutathione, then colonics* to remove the mercury and other poisons from my body. I hasten the process by sweating during workouts and in saunas. I also take supplements such as selenium. To rid myself of aluminum, I drink silica water. I swallow a teaspoon of glycine twice daily to speed urinary glyphosate excretion. I am also starting chlorine dioxide and using a red light from Sauna Space. I wrote this in late 2023, three months after I started, and I am a little better.

Hat makers used mercury in past centuries, and "mad as a hatter" became their stereotype. I have always been a bit quirky, slightly hyper, and prone to anxiety. A psychiatrist friend once informally skewered me with a diagnosis and, as is their religion, recommended a useless, toxic medication. I tried it for a week, then threw it out.

Fortunately, my wife—most of the time—accepts me as I am. Her dental health disasters are much more severe than mine. (Chapter 1).

In Europe, mercury fillings are slowly being phased out. However, many US dentists still use them promiscuously for children and patients on public insurance programs. Amalgams are cheap, easy to place, and profitable.

*I, too, was skeptical at first. I spent two weeks in Germany, getting intravenous medications daily and colon therapy three times a week. Each time, they used a machine to run a liter of water in and out of my colon *every minute for an hour*. Decades of experience detoxing patients with and without colonics prove these work. They eliminate some of the toxins that the IVs mobilize.

Introduction

It is of no consequence to you what other people think of you. What matters is what you think of them. That is how you live your life.

— Gore Vidal

In this era of hospital abuses and the Covid "vaccine," living your life according to the opinions of others can get you killed. In my case, I have been forced to adopt Vidal's attitude because I am under fire. A reviewer wrote, "Your book is a horrible snipe attack on dentists who spend their careers trying to prevent dental problems and keep people healthy. Dentists are good people who would not do anything they knew would hurt anyone." She is correct, and yes, my work is a rabid assault.

But I judge people by what they do and not what they say. Willful ignorance is a scant excuse for anything, least of all criminality. The evidence is clear—most dentistry is toxic and dangerous. Their practices are killing us.

I investigated dentists only after discovering what they did to my health. By the end of this book, you will realize that they have the same effects on you and your family.

I have no delusions about the innocence of MDs and have spent the better part of the last four years exposing them and the rest of the medical industry. Their priority has always been profits and never our health. They have succeeded in turning many of us into lifelong patients dependent on their "care."

The second part of this book, "Judas Dentists Live Inside the Rockefeller Medicine Matrix," explains the dark forces commanding all species of dentists and doctors. We are being pressed into fostering a host of lethal, man-made plagues. Few of us understand that we are playing a part in a vast, networked conspiracy that seeks to kill a lot of us (Chapter 12).

A cabal seized governments worldwide. They used public officials, including the judiciary, as their henchmen and forced the surrender of our sovereignty to their profit machine. Hitler, Stalin, and Mao used dogs and sticks to get victims to capitulate, but today, big tech and the mainstream media use propaganda to compel us to take biohazards. Those unwilling to surrender are shamed and harassed. In the US, we are fortunate not to have been put into "quarantine camps" as happened elsewhere.

The Covid vax is the criminal network's most deadly threat so far. For the first time, they were able to decrease live births and increase disability, chronic illness, and overall deaths. This was documented by insurance data and exposed by Edward Dowd and others (See my last book, *Cassandra's Memo*).

This is a black pill, a bitter insight; understanding it is agonizing. But if you keep your faith through the last chapter, I will put a lightsaber in your hands to wield against the attackers. You need only have the strength to pick it up.

Dentists and doctors commit treason, not just malpractice

They swear the Hippocratic oath, "Put your patients' welfare above your own." It is a binding contract, but nearly all of them dishonor it. When they do, they become accessories to murderous psychopaths (See Chapter 12).

I always thought dentists were somewhat dull colleagues who still deserved respect. But as I studied them, I realized their treachery surpassed any medical specialty (except possibly pediatrics). Make no mistake—I am furious with MDs. What they do is a monstrous net harm. But the dentists... Self-reflection, objective analysis, and patient-first ethics seem outside their considerations.

I interviewed two senior dentists, Dr. Gammal from Australia (Chapter 6) and another from Europe, who requested anonymity. *They independently told me that dental care is closely related to forty percent of diseases in the developed world.* You will soon learn that this is not hyperbole. In less affluent countries, dentistry is less hazardous because it is less "advanced."

We should learn from veterinarians. They are responsible for both their animals' bodies and teeth and are said to look in a horse's mouth first. It is also the best practice to evaluate people. But for humans, the "caregivers" built a Chinese wall between the mouth and the rest of the body. Physicians barely see the mouth, and dentists are not trained to consider systemic disease.

This has been disastrous for patients. For example, oral bacteria have been found in the majority of coronary artery blockages and have been discovered inside Alzheimer's disease brain structures. Also, when mercury dissolves from dental fillings and spreads throughout the body, it persists and causes chronic toxicity.

Dental felonies

Wisdom teeth extraction: Dentists sell this to anyone with a mouth. Their pitch is, "Remove them now and prevent the possibility of removal later if they become impacted." Their websites make the improbable claim that over two-thirds of everyone eventually needs this surgery. Some dentists even claim that premolars, the teeth in front of the molars, should also be pulled out "to make more room in your mouth." See the end of Chapter 2 for more.

This is the same retarded reasoning that gynecologists use to sell ovary removal during hysterectomies "to prevent ovarian cancer." These tumors are rare, and cutting ovaries out leaves women vulnerable to osteoporosis and myriad other diseases of aging. Like wisdom teeth removal, the procedure is a net loss, and like pulling normal teeth, it is easy surgery and easy money. (*Butchered by "Healthcare"* tells that story; word search for "hysterectomy.")

Fluoride: As endorsed by the American Dental Association, more than 90 percent of the US, Canada, and Australia drink water poisoned with fluoride. Most of it comes from lead-contaminated Chinese sources. To conveniently dispose of their waste, chemical producers pay the American Dental Association millions yearly to promote fluoride's supposed benefits. But it is a neurotoxin that, among other hazards, decreases children's IQs. The rest of the world has mostly banned it. (See Chapter 9).

Mercury fillings. This pre-Civil War technology uses one of the most toxic metals known. These are banned in much of the world.

Root canals are the dentists' worst crimes. They involve dead or nearly dead teeth that are drilled out, mummified with toxins and carcinogens, and then left in place to rot. Root canals are always infected and spread bacteria to the rest of the body, destroying or at least compromising the victims' health.

Root canals were repudiated by their inventors over a half-century ago. However, they are so profitable that both general dentists and endodontists, their ethically challenged subspecialty, continue the practice. The heavily referenced *Root Cause* video HERE convicts these "professionals" of assault, malpractice, and incompetence. (If this link is censored, search for a free version. It is available on Rumble currently.)

Titanium implants create related problems.

We are invested in dental lies. Sixty percent of Europeans and somewhat fewer people in the rest of the First World live with embalmed teeth. At least half of US dentists still use mercury fillings, and about half of adults here have them. Around 75 percent of us get our wisdom teeth pulled out. These scams are only possible because none of them is immediately painful. How could our nice dentists be doing all this to us?

To put dentistry in context, meet some traitors

Gutless pediatricians have danced in a conga line for decades, hard-selling vaccines for the manufacturers. No study has compared these against a saline placebo—ever. The result is that Pharma pays our kiddie doctors to mindlessly traffic poisons. It is a brutal assault on those we love most. Over the past 40 years, it caused the US autism rate to rise from 1/10,000 to 1/30. This will tear our society apart unless we ban vaccines and deploy a cure. See the last chapter to learn about that.

Psychiatrists are drug pushers proffering elixirs that they claim cure a thousand ills. Sorry, I exaggerated. Only 450 "diagnoses" are found in their billing bible, the Diagnostic and Statistical Manual of Mental Disorders (DSM). To fabricate these, American Psychiatric Association members—paid handsomely by Pharma—cast votes. These "physicians" claim that "disclosing their financial conflicts of interests" fumigates this bribery.

The psych "diseases" concocted by these shills are expressly designed to be "treated" using pricey patented drugs. Pharma supplies half of the Food And Drug Administration (FDA) budget just as they pay the doctors, so their approval is a rubber stamp. Finally, massive disease-mongering campaigns run by corporate ad agencies convince us to use the purported remedies. Since the drugs are all highly addictive, little persuasion is needed after that.

This "mental health" industry has persuaded over a quarter of Americans (and 80 percent of Danes) to swallow psych drugs. Monthly shots are forced on others. These medications numb us, addict us, and cause violence, suicide, and social dysfunction. None has been proven effective.

The proof of that is that—just like every vaccine—the jackals running big Pharma never ran tests of their pricey nostrums against placebo controls. Studies lacking this vital metric are nonsensical. When the authors publish, they prove their work is a scam, the journal editors admit they are accessories, and the companies confess they are ringleaders in a racketeering conspiracy. The FDA blinds itself because it is paid off. All the people involved are murderers, for the drugs are killers.

Other medical specialties slaughter their patients as well. See *Butchered by "Healthcare"* and Part 2 of this book for more. Prescription drugs cause more US fatalities than any health issue but cancer and heart disease (*Deadly Medicines and Organised Crime: How Big Pharma Has Corrupted Healthcare* by Peter Gøtzsche and, more recently, his updated journal article HERE).

My anonymous expert told me appalling tooth tales

He reported that although most MDs start their training with high ideals, dental school supports no God except money. He went on to say that few dentists check blood pressure or use monitoring devices during sedation. Intravenous drugs may stop breathing, but if there is a monitor, it beeps loudly. The doctor has a chance to pump air into the patient's lungs until he* recovers. Without this, the patient might die.

In my expert's experience, dentists rarely bother to ask their patients about their medical histories. For "real" doctors, the standard of care is to have a specialist—or at least a physician who knows the patient—examine those with health problems before surgery. Dereliction of these basic standards routinely results in disaster.

The expert told me:

A DDS colleague I will call Charles, called to tell me his patient had just died in the chair. I asked him, "What was his medical history?" He replied that he did not know. I learned later that the patient had heart disease.

I then asked Charles what the cardiac monitor showed. He replied he does not use one. This guy charges more than a monitor's cost for every crappy titanium implant he places.

I also asked how many shots of anesthetic with adrenaline he gave the man. He told me that he "lost track." Those of us who remember our most basic training know that excess adrenaline can be fatal, especially for heart patients. We also understand that too much local anesthetic is poisonous.

I told the dentist he was lost and that he should pray. But the family never filed a lawsuit, so no one ever found out that Charles had carelessly killed his patient.

My expert added:

Dentists do not use sterile technique, so their patients periodically get massive infections. When dentists attend operating room training, their carelessness is an embarrassment. The nurses must frequently ask them to re-glove after they thoughtlessly contaminate themselves by touching chairs or tables during surgery.

Since I was a surgical center inspector in my past life, I have heard plenty of stories about physicians making mistakes like these. They sometimes get their licenses revoked.

*A basic grammar lesson for those who think this pronoun should have been "they" or "he/she." As used here, "he" refers to both sexes. If you think otherwise, you believe the conspirators who are blurring the wonderful differences between the sexes.

Part One

Dentists are "healthcare" apostates

Chapter 1
A 🤍 Story About the Star of My Show

Recalled to life.

— Charles Dickens, *A Tale of Two Cities*

Our kindly dentist almost killed my wife, Judy. During her late teens, she had a single front tooth destroyed in an auto accident. So this dentist carved the teeth on either side to support a bridge. When these died, he drilled and mummified them into "root canals." As the years passed, he murdered tooth after tooth, leaving their corpses in her mouth to rot and ultimately support three more bridges. But she always looked great. See Chapter 6 to learn more about this process.

I, too, became a patient of this dentist after I married Judy 35 years ago. I already had seventeen mercury fillings when I met him, so he must have thought I had little left to "work" on. He mostly left me alone.

Four years ago, Judy became progressively sicker over about a year. We consulted more than 20 Kaiser doctors. They were all clue-less, and none of them looked in Judy's mouth or even asked about it.

So I began to study and consult outside physicians. Following their advice, I wrote to the Kaiser docs and directed them to run various tests. Since my letters became part of Judy's chart, the doctors did what I asked. It was soon obvious that Judy had "AL amyloido-sis." Until recently, this was rapidly fatal, but new medications prolong survival.

I asked about using daratumumab, the drug that later stabilized Judy's disease. But the Kaiser oncologist categorically refused to consider it and chided me for my suggestion. He said it was "not the standard of care" and it was "only used by cowboys." So I took her to Stanford. This cost more than $30,000 for two chemo sessions and two doctor visits, one of which was virtual. It saved Judy's life, but she became a dependent, miserable cash cow of for-profit Medi-cine. Throughout her illness, we were forced to hire doctors from outside Kaiser to direct Judy's care.

Among other problems, Judy salivated heavily. All night, every hour, I listened to her nearly choke to death in bed beside me. Since I was formerly a board-certified emergency physician, I understood compromised airways and always feared the worst. But she was always optimistic and did not think it was dangerous.

Judy and I are (reasonably!) open with each other, and I thought I knew (nearly!) everything about her. She was always unwilling to share much about her teeth, and I respected her privacy for decades. But as I learned more about dentistry, I had to find out what was in her mouth.

Her illness was a detective story. The "break in the case" was when we were in Tijuana having my mercury fillings removed. I was sneaky—I asked her to let Dr. Lagos "have a quick look" and "grab an x-ray to be sure everything was OK." When they exited the exam room, Judy was beaming. She told me, "No worries. Everything is fine."

I may have been married last week, but it was not yesterday. I grabbed Lagos by the elbow, pulled him into another room, and closed the door. He knew that I knew the jig was up and admitted that Judy had four (4) root canals. He did not like them any better than I did, but he knew better than to argue with a 69-year-old woman.

Since I had been studying full-time while everyone else was playing, I saw the whole thing immediately. Judy's amyloidosis was caused by abscessed root canals spreading infection and inflammation throughout her body. Dr. Gammal told many stories about breast cancer and other serious diseases going away when root-canalled teeth were taken out. So I knew removing them would create better than even odds of curing her.

Judy is profoundly skeptical, which has served her well. She initially refused to consider that, just this once, I might be right. After all, her mouth did not hurt, and her teeth looked great. I would have to persuade her to cooperate to save her life.

I love Judy dearly and did not want to lose her. Her refusal to believe me made me feel for a month like my head was being held underwater. I coaxed her into reading much of Gammal's book and had her watch the *Root Cause* video. I initially thought I would have to tie her to the couch in front of the TV.

While Judy was balking, I was researching. Becky Dutton (Chapter 11) told me to see a particular European dentist. When Judy finally allowed that she might consider doing something, I put Becky on the phone to work her over.

Next was the flight overseas and six hours of surgery under general anesthesia. The surgeon removed all but one of Judy's teeth, including the infected root canals. The operating room filled with a foul stench because my wife's teeth and gums were abscessed. He said later that her condition would have been fatal soon.

The surgeon cleaned the area, bone-grafted it, and inserted fifteen zirconia ceramic posts to support the new teeth and bridges:

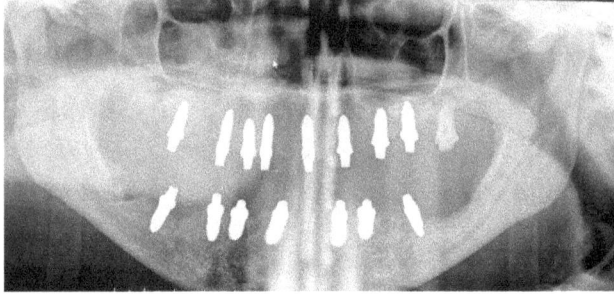

These are biologically inert, and their placement requires specialized skills. Titanium is commonly used, but this causes chronic infections and sheds toxic metals. For more about this, see Chapter 6. Nonfunctional cosmetic teeth were placed in Judy's mouth until the new teeth were inserted three months later.

We stayed a month for the follow-up visits. Judy was instructed to chop up and swallow her food without chewing. She did not like it but adapted and did not lose weight.

Three months after the original surgery, Judy felt fantastic. She had more energy than in years and was starting new projects, which was the best evidence of better health. She also started lifting weights for the first time in four years.

Judy was able to discontinue some of her blood pressure drugs because the infection stress was gone. Her skin was clear of the blemishes that her chronic infection likely caused. The salivation from her inflamed mouth decreased as well.

As I write this, she is getting fitted with her permanent teeth. They are beautiful and stronger than the originals. The process costs half of what it would have in the US, but we nearly had to sell real estate to pay for it. This is not easy for retirees on fixed incomes, but for recalling Judy to life, it is a small price to pay.

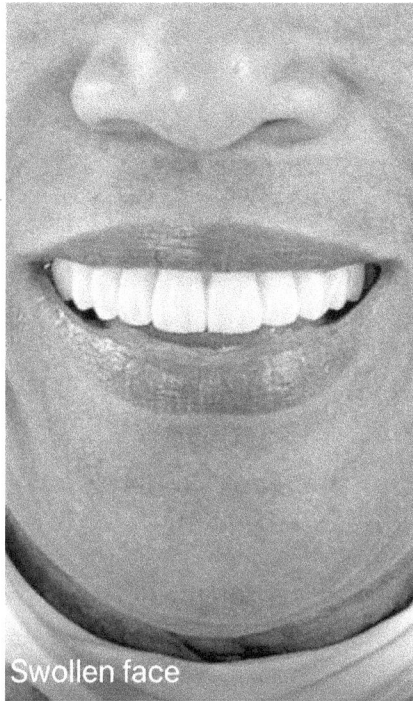

Swollen face

Judy's new teeth, Feb 29, 2024

PS: If you have problems like Judy's, email Becky Dutton (Chapter 11, beckydutton@understandingscoliosis.org), and she will advise you.

PPS: Breast implants, especially silicone ones, cause a similar syndrome known as "breast implant illness (BII)." They are often infected with bacteria and fungi, and the gel they contain is toxic, migrates, and occasionally causes cancer. I interviewed an expert about this HERE.

Chapter 2
I Thought Dentists Were Inferior Animals Before I Learned About Doctors

P sychiatrists, pediatricians, dentists, and every other medical profession are bought-and-paid-for industry shills. For the dentists, exhibit A is dental products, B is fluoridation, and C is mercury amalgams and root canals.

LINK

Before I start bashing dentists, I confess that I was once an acolyte of Jay Geier, one of their marketing gurus (schedulinginsti-tute.com). I attended his conferences with hundreds of dentists and a few cosmetic surgeons to learn about corporate sales. Part of what he did was to teach geeky professionals how to dress, make eye contact, and even keep their offices clean. I learned a lot but spent tens of thousands of dollars. My wife, who was writing the checks, informed me repeatedly that Jay was a fraud.

Exhibit A: Never trust commercial toothpaste or oral care products

In an age when we are hearing rumors about Big Agriculture putting genocidal mRNA bioweapons in our food, worrying about toothpaste, mouthwash, and dentists seems trivial. We might soon be in a scene like the escape from the gulag in the movie *Mad Max Beyond Thunderdome*. Max asks the train conductor, "What's the plan?" He replies, "There ain't no plan... the track ends in four miles."

But even if the apocalypse is nigh, you should learn that holding chemicals in your mouth puts them into your bloodstream nearly as quickly as giving them intravenously. For example, nitroglycerine on your gums immediately relieves chest pain from heart disease. And even though Proctor and Gamble claims their products are "Iconic brands you can trust," thoughtlessly scrubbing them into your mouth pushes whatever corporate marketers cook up directly into your body. Spitting it out does not get rid of it in time.

Since 1997, the FDA has required a warning on every toothpaste tube, "If more than used for brushing is accidentally swallowed, get medical help or contact a poison control center right away." They also said that children under six should only use a pea-sized amount.

Studies implicate mouthwash in head and neck cancers. One common ingredient, chlorhexidine, raises blood pressure. Triclosan, widely used in dentistry, is a pesticide that has been shown to harm kidney function (*Toxic Teeth: How a Biological (Holistic) Dentist Can Help You Cure Cancer, Facial Pain, Autoimmune, Heart, and Other Disease Caused By Infected Gums, Root Canals, Jawbone Cavi-*

tations, and Toxic Metals (2019) by JM Swartz, MD, and YL Wright, MA).

Every corporate concoction is potentially harmful. We know the people selling them prioritize only profits, have little regard for health, and will say anything to increase sales. Likewise, the endorsement of multiple toothpastes by the American Dental Association proves solely that the companies paid for it.

All conventional toothpastes and most fluoride-free "natural" ones have artificial sweeteners. Cyclamate, the first of these fake sugars, was invented in 1937. In 1969, when the annual sales were a billion dollars, studies proved that it caused bladder cancer in rats. The US initially banned it from foods, then took it off the market in 1970. Abbott Laboratories, the owner, petitioned to have it reinstated in the US several times but failed. It is still approved in 130 foreign countries. Saccharin was banned in 1981 for similar issues.

Six artificial sugars are now approved in the US. Xylitol, the alcohol form of xylose sugar, is found in many toothpastes, including some from health food stores. It is a non-nutritive, antiviral, and antibacterial plant sweetener that is naturally present in some berries. My friend and mentor Martha Rosenberg wrote an article about its positive attributes that you may download here.

But like other chemical sweeteners, there are internet claims that xylose causes blood sugar disturbances that contribute to diabetes. A search reveals reports of irritable bowel syndrome, diarrhea, kidney stones, and cancer. Higher doses are said to produce liver failure. The European Union forbids the use of this sugar in soft drinks, and a single piece of xylitol chewing gum can kill small dogs. Whether this is true or simply bad press generated by competitors is unclear.

I do not need to review all the non-nutritive sweeteners to convince you they deserve no place in your body. Most have been implicated in health hazards. These fakes are everywhere—sodas, candies, sports drinks, and energy drinks. Most of us thoughtlessly pound this stuff down every day. I did until recently.

No Pharma or food company's research is trustworthy. For example, saccharine's follow-up studies suggested it did not cause cancer: "Most studies of the other five approved artificial sweeteners have provided no evidence that they cause cancer or other adverse health effects in lab animals."

Do you think the corporations making the money will ever perform real studies on these products? Do we need to waste time looking at other ingredients in commercial oral hygiene products before trashing them?

Alternatives and Solutions

HERE is an article describing seven nontoxic alternatives to commercial toothpaste. These are charcoal, Bentonite clay, baking soda, neem (from the evergreen tree), miswak (twigs of the Salvadora persica tree), and sea salt. (Large particles of salt are rumored to damage tooth enamel.) Another possibility recommended by a reader is Takesumi Supreme charcoal powder.

Here is what I do. After using a Waterpik, I brush my teeth with coconut oil using my Sonicare. I then do "coconut oil pulling," swishing it around my mouth and through my teeth for up to twenty minutes. Since I write all day, this is not socially awkward or time-consuming. It removes residual food particles, inhibits plaque formation, and, in my experience, eliminates the need to floss much. It may be the best tip here if you want to fire your dentist—and who doesn't? Spit it out, but not down the drain, because it can cause blockage. A gallon of Costco coconut oil costs $20.

Mercola recommends putting hydrogen peroxide in your Waterpik reservoir and your mouthwash. To try this, pour some 3% hydrogen peroxide into the Waterpik tank, then fill it with water. You do not need to measure the exact quantity because most people tolerate it even at 50 percent strength (1.5%). I use a teaspoon of the 50:50 mix for mouthwash, and it foams satisfyingly.

I use the cheap Costco brand, but HERE is one that is food-grade. This process can make infected gums pink and healthy in a few weeks, but it irritates some. Switch to coconut oil pulling or try quarter strength if this happens. Note: the optimal use of peroxide might be for limited periods.

This is more than a cosmetic issue; the bacteria in dental plaque and diseased gums spread to coronary artery blockages and many other places in your body. THIS excellent podcast explains.

I also use chlorine dioxide (CD) mouthwash. You can get a commercial product from FrontierPharm, and HERE is an affiliate link you can use to order it. You get a discount, and I donate the commissions to charities promoting CD use. I have more about this in the Epilogue. I will show you how to make your CD later in this book.

Weston Price, a dentist whose work survives at the Weston A Price Foundation, studied tribes in remote third-world areas and found that the ones who ate no refined sugar or wheat had no tooth decay. After trade started and they began consuming these, the tribe people began to have tooth decay. After traders stopped bringing these foods to one remote island, Price visited and found signs that their cavities had started to heal. His Weston Price Foundation promotes animal-based diets, hates root canals, and educates us about other health issues.

I try to strictly avoid sugar and bread, but it is not easy.

Similar chemicals in deodorants should also be avoided

Almost all contain aluminum. This is toxic and has been closely tied to Alzheimer's. In the early 2000s, it was added to vaccines after most of the mercury was removed. It is best to avoid it by using those with none, such as the "Life Doesn't Stink" roll-on.

Baking soda is even better and costs about two cents daily (Arnie at Liar's World Substack gave me this idea). Use a volume of about three or four American quarters, moisten it with water, and apply.

Caveat: using too much causes skin irritation. Some only need it every other day.

Since it is hard to get too much magnesium, I sometimes use a magnesium-based roll-on deodorant. I poured my Colgate mouth-wash into the toilet and filled the bottle with a 25 % hydrogen perox-ide-water mouthwash mix (.75 percent). Tom's toothpaste contains xylose, but I sometimes use it anyway. I keep my dog Tucker out of the bathroom to keep him safe. When I checked my Sonicare tooth-brush with an EMF meter, I was relieved to find nothing.

Exhibit B: fluoridation summary (see Chapter 8 as well)

In America, phosphate fertilizer companies dispose of their industrial waste fluoride by putting it into our drinking water. These companies subsidize the American Dental Association with millions of dollars every year. In return, they rabidly promote the fluoride benefits for teeth and general health.

Swartz (cited above) writes, "The more [fluoride] is used, the greater the damage to the central nervous system [brain].[145] It should never be used in dentistry or any product. Putting it in drinking water is criminal... It does not prevent tooth decay. It causes dental problems over time." Fluoride has been proven to significantly lower children's IQs.

The best way to understand these issues is through the Fluoride Action Network. They are pursuing fluoridators through the US federal courts. In a recent victory, the judge on the case released a comprehen-sive summary of the expert science indicting fluoride. It cited irrefutable studies proving pregnant mothers' high urine fluoride levels were related causally to profoundly depressed children's IQs. Biden officials, including Rachel Levine, transgender admiral and later Secretary of Health, are managing the litigation on the wrong side. (Update HERE.)

Seventy percent of US communities are victimized by fluoride, but most of the rest of the world has banned it. In Europe, for example, 97% of the countries choose not to fluoridate drinking water. If you live in the USA and you do not want stupid children, you must rid your water of fluoride using filters, distilled water, or reverse osmosis systems such as Culligan's.

Water fluoridation by country (Wiki).

Postscript: About a quarter of prescription drugs have toxic fluoride structures, including:

✪ Statins (Lipitor, Crestor, etc.)

✪ Anti-inflammatories (some steroids and NSAIDs)

✪ Antacids (Prevacid)

✪ Antidepressants and antipsychotics (including nearly all SSRIs like Prozac)

✪ Some antibiotics (Levaquin/Cipro)

✪ Some antifungals (Fluconazole)

Avoid them if you can.

Exhibit C: Amalgam "silver" dental fillings and root canals

Amalgams are a pre-Civil War technology that should have been outlawed long ago. Half of US dentists acknowledge this and never use it because of mercury hazards. Amalgams are inexpensive and more profitable for dentists than newer technologies. Ignorant or unscrupulous practitioners often place them in poor patients who use Medicaid federal insurance. Many dental schools and the American Dental Association still refuse to acknowledge mercury's dangers and continue to promote amalgam fillings against a mountain of established science.

The following is also from *Toxic Teeth*.

Amalgam ("silver") fillings are a mixture of several metals, one of which is mercury. Nickel, lead, aluminum, and cadmium are also used in the alloys. These all tend to leech out of the fillings and are absorbed into the body's tissues. [Other sources say these often also contain tin, zinc, and sometimes copper, the most toxic of the last three.]

[These] "silver" fillings are made up of 50% mercury, which [causes] health problems... Mercury fillings represent the largest mercury exposure to people worldwide. Dr. Friberg, the chief advisor of the World Health Organization, insists that there is no safe mercury exposure level. Mercury is one of the most toxic naturally occurring substances in the world.

Medical professionals realize this. If a mercury thermometer was still being used in a hospital and it broke, the whole floor would be closed down, and the hazmat team would come in to clean it up. A dental filling has about fifty times as much mercury as a thermometer. Mercury exposure is deadly, affecting the way you think and feel. [83] [84]

If you have a mouth that contains one or more fillings made with mercury (amalgam or silver) fillings, you are constantly exposed to toxicity.[85] When you chew or brush your teeth, mercury is released from the fillings and goes into your body's tissues. This happens from the very first day the mercury filling is placed into your mouth by a dentist, until it is removed.

There is no safe way to place an amalgam filling. Mercury amalgam is the absolute worst material being used to fill cavities. Careful barrier techniques are crucial when removing mercury to protect patient, doctor, and staff from mercury exposure during the procedure. Because the fillings do not last, they must be replaced repeatedly. However, safety in removing mercury amalgams is usually not a priority in most dental offices. This causes toxic exposure to the

*patient, the dentist, dental personnel, and anyone in the office. The
media is unaware of this problem.*

*Mercury vapor is released from amalgams[86] when you chew[87]
and crosses right through the blood-brain barrier. The more mercury
you have in your mouth, the more mercury you have in your brain[88]
and kidneys.[89] [90] It may take some time for symptoms to present
themselves as the mercury slowly builds up in the body. Early symptoms like fatigue, difficulty sleeping, anxiety, and depression may not
be easily recognized as being associated with the amalgam fillings.
Mercury from fillings can create many common symptoms, including
depression, anxiety, chronic fatigue,[91] chronic headaches, digestive
upsets, depression, and memory problems.[92]*

*Mercury toxicity in a pregnant woman and also in the father[93]
can cause problems in the unborn child.[94] [95] Mercury causes
destruction of your cells[96] and leaky membranes.[97] Mercury
vapor causes damage to both sciatic and optic nerves [98] and nasal
sinuses. Breathing in the mercury vapor takes the mercury straight into
the brain,[99] damaging the lungs.[100] [101]*

*Amalgams are a massive source of environmental pollution.[102]
The dental industry dumps about 4.4 tons of mercury into the planet
annually. Mercury doesn't just come from coal-fired energy plants. It
comes from dentists who keep putting it into people's mouths. Imagine
the enormous amount of mercury that is released into the environment
when someone who has mercury fillings dies and is cremated.[103]*

More:

Swartz had dental care every six months his entire life. No cavities were seen except during a brief period at college when a dentist
mysteriously discovered a dozen and filled them with mercury amalgams. I had the same experience when I was about ten—I had 17
amalgams placed over two years. No one discovered other problems
in my mouth before or since besides him. Swartz and my mother
trusted these people. Behind closed doors, dentists call this "drill, fill,
and bill."

Dr. Mercola had two dozen mercury fillings installed during his youth under similar circumstances. He had them removed later, but that work was done by a conventional dentist who did not use barrier methods or a vapor evacuation system. This damaged Mercola's kidneys.

"Biological" dentists specialize in removing and replacing the outdated, hazardous metals in patients' mouths. These include root canals, which frequently contain mercury and are also sources of chronic, usually asymptomatic, infections.

"Cavitations" adjacent to dental appliances appear lighter on the X-rays and are usually infected. The problem typically starts when the ligament that attached the tooth to the bone is left in place when a tooth is extracted. These must be thoroughly drilled out. This produces symptom relief in about eighty percent and often improves health dramatically (References: Swartz above and Robert Gammal's book, see Chapter 6).

Swartz advises choosing a dentist who uses the Huggins methodology and is certified by Hal Huggins. They know that if the mouth is unhealthy, the rest of the body cannot be healthy.

Chew On This... But Don't Swallow by Grube and Vazquez-Tibau (2022) is a similar reference with other stunning stories. One of the authors, a dentist with decades of occupational mercury exposure, had her blood work checked during a holistic dentist conference and was diagnosed with lymphoma. After her root canals and amalgams were removed, she was cured. Her fatigue and lifelong concentration problems disappeared as well. She notes:

✪ Amalgams that start with 54% mercury contain 28% twenty-five years later.

✪ Norway, Denmark, and Sweden have banned the use of dental mercury.

✪ In 2018, the European Union banned mercury for pregnant women, breastfeeding women, and children under 15.

✪ Huggins's training is the standard for biological dentists.

Yoho comment as this was written: I am 69 years old and have seventeen amalgams. My blood mercury level is zero, but this is common with mercury toxicity because it gets stored in the brain, muscles, and other tissues. My fillings seem stable, but they are only designed to last twenty-five years. Most of mine are over fifty years old.

My traditional dentist advised me that removing and replacing them with mercury-free materials might be riskier than leaving them in. However, I have a worsening undiagnosed neurological condition, so I decided to get all seventeen removed.

References

Mercola's dental podcasts:

✪ "Mercury Awareness Week" is HERE.

✪ It's all in your mouth" is HERE.

✪ "Mercury free dentistry week" is HERE.

✪ HERE is an interview with Dr. Thomas Levy about how tooth disease causes heart disease and cancer.

✪ HERE is a video testimonial from Stacy Case, a news anchor whose multiple sclerosis disappeared when her mercury amalgams were removed.

Parting shot: Dr. Mercola about wisdom tooth extraction

HERE is the article. His summary:

✪ Estimates suggest that five million people have their wisdom teeth removed each year, and more than half of this may be unnecessary. According to a 2005 Cochrane Review, "Prudent decision-making, with adherence to specified indicators for removal, may reduce the number of surgical procedures by 60% or more."

✪ There are no proven health benefits to removing wisdom teeth that are not causing problems.

✪ Many oral health experts recommend extracting wisdom teeth only if they are growing at an odd angle, causing pain, are affected by tooth decay, are impacting other teeth, or are causing inflammation.

✪ Extracting wisdom teeth is not risk-free, even if you are young. Complications associated with the surgery include poor wound healing, infection, dry socket, pain, uncontrolled bleeding, and nerve injury resulting in numbness around the mouth and face.

✪ Opioid addiction is another hidden risk because most oral surgeons prescribe opioids for post-surgical pain. Research shows that a combination of ibuprofen and acetaminophen* works better than opioids for pain following wisdom tooth extraction. Avoid opioids at all costs.

Chapter 3
Scott Schroeder, DPM: Dental and Orthopedic Metals Can Make You Sick

T hese and other metals in the body create an electrical battery effect with dental amalgams that release toxic mercury.

LINK

Dr. Schroeder's interview includes patient audio testimonials about how they improved after removing metals from their bodies. He wrote:

I have placed thousands of metallic implants in my patients over my 30-year foot and ankle surgeon career. I didn't ask many questions about metal allergies or reactions early in my practice. But when my partner placed titanium alloy screws during my wife's bunion surgery, I started paying attention.

After the surgery, she had burning, shooting pains every night for four months. She could not even put her foot under the covers and went to bed each night with an ice pack to calm her foot down enough to sleep. When the hardware was taken out, her pain vanished. This was 16 years ago, and it opened my eyes. We learned subsequently that my wife was allergic to the aluminum and nickel present in her titanium alloy screws. These also contained vanadium.

II presented "Systemic Effects of Metal Allergies" to the FDA in 2019. My cases included an engineer in his forties who became paralyzed for 10-12 hours each day shortly after I placed eight 2.0 mm screws into his feet. When he returned for a separate issue four years later, I operated on one of his feet and noticed swelling where the screws were. So, I removed them because of a possible nickel allergy.

When the patient returned for his second post-op visit, he finally told me the paralysis story. He said he had been immobilized for more than ten hours a day, but immediately after I removed the screws, this decreased to three hours a day. He had been seen at Mayo Clinic several times, and they told him, "You are going to be in a wheelchair the rest of your life, and eventually, your wife will have to put you in a nursing home." So, I tested for metal allergies using the "MELISA-optimized lymphocyte transformation assay." It was done at a German lab founded by Dr. Vera Stejskal, a Swedish immuno-toxicologist and inventor of the test.

This showed that the engineer was allergic to nickel and palladium. We learned that the gold crowns in his mouth were 26% palladium and that he also had a titanium alloy screw in his knee. When we removed the screw, he had a minor improvement, but the day his last gold crown was removed from his mouth, his paralysis disappeared and has not returned. That was several years ago.

I have seen many other patients who have had stunning health improvements after I removed metal from their bodies. I have to admit that I had placed most of it!

I have been presenting about this around the world since 2015. I have lectured in Australia, New Zealand, London, Turkey, and the US. Many top researchers and physicians became my mentors and colleagues. When I spoke in London, the Queen's Orthopedist who lectured after me bought my wife and me drinks that night.

Before Dr. Stejskal passed on from breast cancer, she had been primarily working with European surgeons and dentists. They had many cases where the chronic pain associated with a total hip or knee implant would go away after the removal of dental metals. I was intrigued but skeptical and started asking more questions about patients with multiple metals in their bodies. I began seeing patterns.

To learn more, I am working with engineers who specialize in "body galvanic corrosion." Yesterday, the hospital ethics committee approved our study of patients with various symptoms relieved by explanting metals. This is a combined effort of the University of Victoria and the University of British Columbia. I am an adjunct faculty member working with a professor at the University of Victoria.

Scott describes two separate issues:

✪ Allergy to orthopedic metals.

✪ Metal orthopedic implants create a battery effect or a current with mercury-filled dental amalgams.

Metal implants are now ubiquitous. The most commonly recognized allergies to their components involve nickel, cobalt, chromium, and bone cement, which can be aluminum-based. Practicing orthopedists like my co-interviewer Jeff Martin and MR, another senior orthopedist, have vast experience. They say these are rare, and MR adds:

I occasionally see metal allergies, but we don't know how common they are. We occasionally consult an allergist before or after surgery as required. The patient usually thinks of this issue and asks us about it. I have not seen dramatic cures after metal removal for severe symptoms such as paralysis.

Ways to check for allergies: Sending blood to Germany for the MELISA test may not be necessary. Allergists can place skin patches that have these substances on them. If a rash is seen when they take them off a few days later, the patient is considered allergic to whatever was on the patch. Nickel allergy is the most common; five to twelve percent of the population has it. Taping a nickel coin to the inner thigh and checking for a rash under it in a day or two is a simple test for this.

Some practitioners use blood, urine, breath, hair, saliva, and even stool analysis to evaluate mercury toxicity. For chronic exposures—which are the majority—these tests are usually negative and an unneeded expense. Most authorities recommend the removal of any amalgams and, if possible, all orthopedic devices. If the patient improves, that is all anyone cares about.

Treatment: After the amalgams are out, the exposure declines and the body starts clearing toxins. However, most cannot be easily removed because they are embedded in tissues such as muscles and the brain. Symptomatic improvement, if it happens, can take months to years.

Traditional chelating agents such as intravenous dimercaprol (BAL) or dimercapto succinic acid (DMSA) bind metals and are reputed to facilitate their urinary elimination.

The top experts recommend intravenous phosphatidylcholine (PC), folinic acid, and glutathione to remove metals. In Chapter 11, Becky Dutton discusses how the traditional chelating agents above may damage kidneys.

According to her authorities, oral glutathione is poorly absorbed. Oral phosphatidylcholine is available in a syrup form from Body bio.com.

Note:

As you work through this book, you will realize dentists work in a profoundly toxic environment. I do not envy them. Swartz (Chapter 2) says that dental amalgams contain over fifty percent volatile mercury:

Reports and research are consistent that these fillings emit mercury vapors. Research demonstrates that dental mercury amalgams expose dental professionals, dental staff, dental patients, and/or fetuses to releases of mercury vapor, mercury-containing particulate, and/or other forms of mercury contamination. Mercury vapor is released from dental mercury amalgam fillings at higher rates during brushing, cleaning, clenching of teeth, chewing, etc., and mercury is also known to be released during the placement, replacement, and removal of dental mercury amalgam fillings.

Other references

To learn about mercury and how to avoid it.

✪ *Mercury-Free: A clear path that guides you and our planet back to good health* by Teresa Franklin, PhD and James Hardy, DMD (2021)

✪ The Heavily Metalled Podcast EP06 Miraculous Surgical Cases, Metal Allergies and Galvanism with Dr. Scott Schroeder, DPM, FACFAS

✪ Dr Scott Schroeder's testimony - FDA Immunology Devices Panel Meeting Day 1 (2019)

✪ See the International Academy of Oral Medicine and Toxicology (IAOMT) website HERE to learn how dentists can remove them safely. Here are a few main points:

- Each room where mercury fillings are removed must have a high-volume air filtration system.
- Face shields, hair/head coverings, and protective gowns and covers for the dentist, dental personnel, and the patient.
- Either a properly-sealed, respiratory-grade mask rated to capture mercury or a positive pressure, properly-sealed mask providing air or oxygen must be worn by the dentist and all dental personnel in the room.

- External air or oxygen delivered via a nasal mask to ensure the patient does not inhale mercury vapor or amalgam particulate during the procedure. A nasal cannula is acceptable if the patient's nose is completely covered with an impenetrable barrier.
- A dental dam made with non-latex nitrile material must be placed and properly sealed in the patient's mouth.
- During amalgam filling removal, the dentist must utilize an oral aerosol vacuum near the operating field (i.e., two to four inches from the patient's mouth) to mitigate mercury exposure.
- The amalgam needs to be sectioned into chunks and removed in as large of pieces as possible using a small diameter carbide drill.

Parting shots

#1. Dentists shamelessly advertise their worst crimes

The following is from one of their websites:

Are Root Canals Safe? We're here to reassure you that modern root canals are not what you may imagine them to be. In fact, 97% of root canals are successful procedures, according to the National Center for Biotechnology Information (NCBI). Plus, 85% of teeth fixed by a root canal last a lifetime.

Although some dentists are ashamed of their actions, those who understand what their specialty is doing seldom repent publicly for fear of retaliation. This can cost them their licenses in the UK and parts of the US. Like me, those who speak up typically wait until after they retire.

Becky Dutton received the following confessional letter from a dentist. I know from experience how painful this is.

I am reading your website with great interest and, if I am completely honest, a feeling of deep guilt and unease having inflicted patients, friends, and family with dental amalgams over a period of 30 years. As dentists, we really were brainwashed into believing that mercury, in the form of amalgam fillings, was completely safe.

My own chronic ill health led me to early retirement in 2015 and to the start of my research into the microbiome, my previously undiagnosed parasitic infection, bad bugs and, of course, heavy metals. Two years ago, I had all my amalgam fillings removed by a holistic dentist who followed the correct guidelines.

Many thanks for creating your website. It has been a mine of eye-opening information.

#2. A few physicians step into the light as well

Paul Thomas and Ken Stoller are pediatricians who disavowed vaccines. Paul interviewed Ken in THIS fantastic podcast.

Psychiatric drugs are highly addictive, universally destructive, and divorced from even the ruined science of the rest of healthcare. I have never heard a psychiatrist other than Peter Breggin or Thomas Szasz repudiate his specialty. These "doctors" have spent their careers running the wrong way down a one-way street. Flipping their minds to rationality is almost impossible.

Scott Schroeder has spent the last decade spreading the word about the health damages of metals. He knows he caused a lot of it.

Plastic and cosmetic surgeons who confess that breast implants are a net harm are practically unheard of. I know only three: Dr. Khan, Dr. Feng, and me. I am retired, but the first two specialize in removing implants with the surrounding scar intact and in one piece. This arduous *en bloc* excision offers the best chance of curing breast implant illness, a syndrome of symptomatic silicone toxicity and the accompanying infections. Check the surgeons' Facebook pages to hear their patients' stories.

Chapter 4
Terri Franklin, Ph.D. Replaced Her Amalgams With Metal-Free Composites

She is the co-author of *Mercury Free*, a book about the horrific health problems associated with implanted metals and how holistic dentists are removing them.

LINK

The following quotes are from *Mercury-Free* by Teresa Franklin, Ph.D. and James Hardy, DMD (2021):

What makes [mercury} amalgam scrap? If it is not in the tooth, it is called scrap. Environmental agencies must be contacted for proper

*disposal methods of that little piece of amalgam that didn't go in the
tooth. If amalgam is unsafe to put in the trash can, how can it be safe in
the mouths and bodies of an estimated 100 million Americans, which
translates to 1/3 of the population? It is not safe, and in fact, based on
a conservative estimate in a population-based trial, over 67 million
Americans exceed the safety exposure level set by the EPA*

*The World Health Organization (WHO) studied mercury expo-
sure to humans from air, water, food, and amalgam fillings and
concluded that the largest source of exposure was dental amalgams.
The WHO also concluded that there was no safe minimum dose of
mercury. "Symptoms are known to occur, at least among some of the
population, at every level of exposure 97,281."*

*Mercury has been banned from interior and exterior latex paint in
the US. Mercury has also been banned in many pesticides. Mercury
has been banned from eyedrops, batteries, smoke detectors, children's
toys, from most vaccines, and its use in thermometers and thermostats
is being drastically reduced and will soon be nonexistent. Other
mercury products, such as mercurochrome and calomel, have been
banned altogether. Mercury use has been prohibited for a reason -
because it is highly toxic. But....explain why mercury has still not been
banned in the most personal environment, the mouth. It makes one
wonder who has the most powerful lobby in Washington DC: the paint
industry, the pesticide industry, or the ADA?*

Dr. Franklin had all four health problems that people can get
with dental appliances:

✪ Metal allergies

✪ Mercury toxicity

✪ A battery effect between the implanted metals causes amalgams to release mercury

✪ Chronic infection

As she gradually figured out what was happening, she started
insisting on proper treatments despite denial and foot-dragging by
her dentists and doctors. Orthopedists are paid poorly for screw

removal, and dentists are brainwashed by the American Dental Association (ADA) to ignore amalgams.

Her health progressively improved over several years as Dr. Teri had her dental appliances removed and replaced with modern "composite" materials. One of her experiences was the drainage of a chronic, nearly asymptomatic abscess that was invisible on a "cone beam" dental X-ray. A globule of mercury was found inside, and the process was shockingly stinky. Another time, patch testing of her skin proved that she had allergies to the metals in her orthopedic implants. Her local orthopedists told her she was crazy, so she flew across the country to get these taken out by Scott Schroeder. She improved dramatically.

Dr. Franklin emphasizes that testing is helpful only for metal *allergies*. None of the available assays for suspected mercury *toxicity* make the diagnosis unless they are highly positive. If they show nothing, mercury might still be hidden in your body. Only after you take out your amalgams and improve can you be sure you have a problem.

X-rays of abscesses, such as her smelly one, typically show signs of the problem but are often read as normal by dentists, who have limited radiology knowledge. Nearly everyone improves dramatically after abscess drainage.

If you have more than one type of metal implanted in your body, an electrical flow is created between them. These cause amalgams to vaporize mercury, which is immediately absorbed into other areas of the body, including the adjacent brain. During surgery, Dr. Schroeder checks for these currents using an electric meter.

Here are a few excerpts from Dr. Franklin's book:

The Food and Drug Administration (FDA) took tuna fish off our grocery shelves when it had only one ppm of mercury. I remembered the Minamata Bay disaster in Japan. The people there ate fish containing mercury, and they suffered high numbers of birth defects, mental retardations, cerebral palsies, and premature deaths directly related to ingesting fish contaminated with mercury.7 So [my question is] "If our government removes tuna fish from stores with only one ppm mercury, how is it even remotely safe to put 700,000 times that much in our patients' teeth and allow them to chew on it for years?"

The mouth is the harshest environment for any material; no material there is considered permanent.

It is nearly impossible to determine how one might feel without a toxic substance without removing it if it has been part of one's life for so long.

Since 1984, numerous scientific articles have been published providing evidence that dentists and their staff have greater neurological, neurobehavioral, kidney, and other disorders and deficits than nondental workers. As we would expect from the insidious nature of mercury, symptoms continue for years and manifest themselves in such a way that one might not even suspect a link. For example, psychosomatic symptoms, problems with memory, concentration, fatigue, and sleep disturbance were all shown to be significantly greater in a study comparing dental assistants with other medical assistants. The video "Is there poison in your mouth," summarizes some of the mercury problems.

The ADA's response to the above, which it still stands by today, was to issue a "Special Report" stating that it is improper and unethical for a dentist to remove amalgams from a non-allergic patient based on the dentist's imperative to remove toxic substances from the patient's body.

Many of my patients have requested amalgam removal for cosmetic reasons or as a hedge against future mercury-related problems. They did not sense any ill effects from having amalgams in their mouths for 25 or more years. But, when the amalgams were replaced, many of these folks noticed unexpected health improvements. Some say their memory improved. Some noticed that they could think more clearly. Others report more energy. Still others report feeling calmer. In more rigorous studies, my general observations have been replicated.

If amalgams have been in your mouth for ten years or longer, be prepared for some issues to be exposed upon removal. There is a 50% failure rate on amalgams that are ten years or older. That means that after around ten years, 50% of them break, fall apart and/or have decay underneath. In some cases, the decay could be significant. Some patients' decay may have progressed to the point that a root canal surgery may be needed.

A study that followed close to 400 people for nearly three years showed a strong link between the presence of amalgam and extra workdays missed. The number of days missed from work was compared the year before amalgam removal and one and two years afterward. The results indicate a 30% drop in sick days two years after amalgam removal.127 What would be the savings in the U.S. of a 30% drop in sick leave among workers? Not to mention, improved morale and productivity while at work and ...improved smiles.

Mercury exposure has been related to MS, cancer, infant death, high blood pressure, low fertility, arrhythmias, thyroid disorders, rheumatoid arthritis, inflammatory bowel disease, chronic fatigue, fibromyalgia, and neurological and psychological disease.

One hundred million amalgam fillings are still placed in Americans' mouths each year, which is the greatest source of environmental and human exposure to mercury. US dentists use 16 tons of mercury a year, and half of it is disposed of improperly.

To prepare to get your amalgams out, [look at the protocols at the IAOMT website, IAOMT.org]. You'll want to be sure your dentist has what Dr. James and I call the 'internal mercury shield' before you start the removal process.

Dr. Franklin says, "I prefer to call the ADA the Amalgam Dental Association."

Dentists who belong to The International Academy of Oral Medicine and Toxicology (IAOMT) clean these problems up

Although there are about 700,000 dentists worldwide, only 1400 of them are IAOMT members. From their website HERE:

[We are] a global network of dentists, health professionals, and scientists who research the biocompatibility of dental products, including the risks of mercury fillings, fluoride, root canals, and jawbone osteonecrosis. We are a non-profit organization and have been dedicated to our mission of protecting public health and the environment since we were founded in 1984.

We accomplish our mission by funding and promoting relevant research, accumulating and disseminating scientific information, investigating and promoting non-invasive scientifically valid therapies, and educating medical and dental professionals, policy makers, and the general public. The IAOMT has a federal tax-exempt status as a non-profit organization under section 501(c)(3) of the Internal Revenue Code, with Public Charity Status 509(a)(2).

Our work is crucial because there is an alarming lack of professional, policy maker, and public awareness about dangerous dental products that are harming humans and the environment on a massive scale. To help change this dire situation, IAOMT members have been expert witnesses about dental products and practices before the US Congress, the US Food and Drug Administration (FDA), Health Canada, the Philippines Department of Health, the European Commission Scientific Committee on Emerging and Newly Identified Health Risks, and other government bodies around the globe. Additionally, the IAOMT is an accredited member of the United Nations Environment Programme (UNEP)'s Global Mercury Partnership and was involved in the negotiations leading to UNEP's Minamata Convention on Mercury.

My reactions as I wrote

I started researching after Debbie Butler pushed me into the pool. Her story is below. I read three books, listened to podcasts, checked references, and interviewed guests.

Teri believes that since the ADA controls dentists, they are nearly blameless. I disagree. Learning about these people shocked me at least as much as finding out about my wretched colleagues. My theory is that, like pediatricians, they are timid, which makes them easily corrupted.

I am (almost) at a loss for words.

My dentist counted seventeen amalgams. When installed, these were 54 percent mercury. About half passes into the rest of the body over twenty-five years. Mine are much older, so I have eaten a lot of mercury.

My "panorex" X-ray is below.

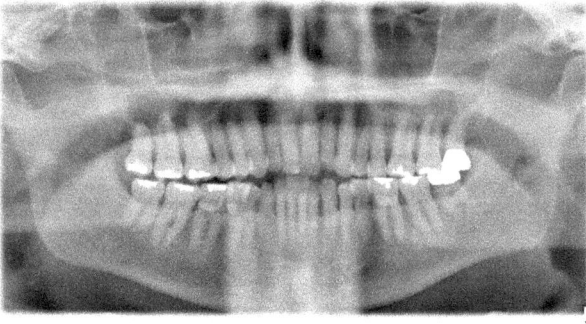

I realize now that my tremor and lifelong low-grade anxiety are likely due to mercury toxicity. My symptoms worsened after my recent shoulder replacements. This must have created electrical effects that more rapidly mobilized the metal.

I am having all seventeen removed and replaced with white "composites." This material is biologically inert. However, it is expensive, more difficult to use, and less profitable for dentists. Once the mercury source is gone, some of my symptoms may gradually clear, but chronic cases like mine may not improve. Wish me luck.

Postscript #1: Mercury detoxification using zeolite

Zeolites are synthetic microporous structures that are available on Amazon. Terri Franklin, her co-author, some IAOMT dentists, and many other sources recommend these. Kerri Rivera, a world expert on the detoxification of autistic children, says that zeolite works if you use the right brand (Chapter 15).

However, Becky Dutton, who has observed hundreds of patients in mercury detox over many years, says that zeolite is not a good chelator and cites this REFERENCE. I could only find it on the Wayback Machine, so it was suppressed. It quotes recognized expert Boyd Haley, professor of chemistry at the University of Kentucky. He writes that zeolite redistributes rather than removes mercury:

[Zeolite] does not significantly remove mercury from an aqueous solution. ... it seems very unlikely that [this] water insoluble material would have any direct effect on removing mercury from cells, mito- chondria, or the brain... How exactly will a non-water soluble material like zeolite cause urinary mercury excretion as shown in previous studies? If the negative charges on the insoluble zeolite really did bind mercury, it should take it out via the fecal route. ... this looks very much like many previous "miracle mercury cures" that just takes a lot of money from the unsuspecting parents looking for any help for their child... but this data was never published in a decent journal...

Zeolites contain high levels of aluminum, a heavy metal. Although the zeolite salespeople talk about how the aluminum in their product is "caged", hair tests done by parents found that aluminum levels spiked.

Haley was involved with developing a related product, so he may have a conflict of interest.

Dutton also privately surveyed six experts in preparation for this book. All had doubts about zeolite. Chris Exley, the "Aluminum

Man," wrote to her: "I would never take [a zeolite]; they have neither been shown to be effective for aluminium in a clinical trial nor indeed to be safe for human consumption. My advice is to avoid."

The sales pitch is that you can buy this product and do it yourself. Since there are pitfalls, an experienced expert should help with any detox process. Many of them recommend safer and more effective methods than zeolite.

Theodore Sturgeon famously said, "Ninety percent of everything is crap." This was from the 1950s, and things are far worse today. Controversy is a sign that something stinks, so I am skeptical of commercial products like these.

Postscript #2: How Debbie Butler took charge of her health

In February 2014, I had my right knee replaced. When I was walking with a cane on the third day following surgery, my tibia split from the knee down. The surgeons operated again and inserted a metal rod. From then on, I needed a walker everywhere I went.

In June 2021, our vehicle was hit by another car, and my right femur broke just above the knee. The surgeons placed a second rod in my leg and replaced the first total knee with a new one. The next day, I could walk up and down steps for the first time in seven years. For 2 1/2 months, I had a spectacular recovery. Unfortunately, I developed an abscess in the anchor tooth of a three-tooth permanent bridge and— worse—had a root canal placed there.

I have been going downhill ever since. I feel pins and needles and have a loss of feeling in both legs. Walking has been difficult. My mouth is numb. I have joint pain, and 90% of my hair has fallen out. I have spent tens of thousands of dollars on functional doctors, naturopaths, and holistic physicians without improvement.

In April 2023, I read Dr. Yoho's Substack post about the metals in vaccines. Mark Kennard from New Zealand wrote a comment about his experience with his orthopedic implants, and the story sounded similar to mine. When I spoke to him, he referred me to Dr. Scott Schroeder, who was nice enough to chat with me for over an hour. I realized that I had likely been suffering from metal reactions since 2014.

I plan to remove as much metal as possible from my body, starting with my mouth. I will tell Dr. Yoho what happens as I go through the process.

The end of the Epilogue tells how Deb cured herself. Spoiler: Getting rid of the metals helped, but she was diagnosed with Lyme disease during the process. So she treated herself with chlorine dioxide and is now "a hundred times better."

Chapter 5
Intermission: Worry less

Today's greatest challenge is to be patient and calm and avoid being intimidated by the psyops. The following will help you throw the garbage out of your mind.

* * *

YOHO'S REALITY RULES
#1. Basic principles:

- Those with the gold make the rules, so learning the funding source explains a lot.
- Lying and damaging others is a drive like sex for psychopaths. Never underestimate your ability to be fooled by them, for they do not telegraph duplicity like ordinary people (Chapter 2, Cassandra's Memo).

#2. Identify what is true.

- Believe your eyes, experience, and intuition, which is the sum of logic and emotions. Have confidence in your discernment powers and take little on faith or authority.
- If a source contains explanations you do not understand, it can generally be cast off as false. Legal arguments often fall into this category. Some technical science fields that require decades of experience must be judged by assessing the person telling the tale.

#3. Use simple heuristics to unearth liars:

- If one of our "colleagues" is all over YouTube, Facebook, or Instagram, he is part of a bowel movement, not the Freedom Movement. Judge us on what stays up and what gets censored. I am a small animal, but the jackals take down everything I put up on social media within 30 minutes.
- "Anybody carrying water for archons, demons, alien invasions, or part-man, part-machine cyborg warriors is either a moron or a paid shill" (Polymath Paul).
- Be suspicious of those who combine hysteria and apocalyptic religion.
- Crediting powerful, previously unknown technology to psychopaths replaces our reasoning powers with atavistic fears about magic.
- Events that are light-years of distance or eons of time away from us are science fiction. Thinking about them is not a practical approach that yields insights or action plans for today.
- The future is unknowable, and predictions are often psyops (Thanks, M!).
- Clues from cancel culture: What is forbidden to be debated isn't true; if debate of a subject is illegal, it is an obvious lie. —Alan Sabrosky

Telling the truth to yourself and others is your highest value. You must ignore stories if they fail the above tests or are supported only by speculative or circumstantial evidence. If your spider sense activates, assume you are being lied to unless you have overwhelming evidence to the contrary.

If you get fooled, trust your intuition once more. Aurelius wrote, "Don't fear the future. You will face it, if that is your fate, armed with the same ruling reason that guides you in the present."

Aurelius again: "Don't become disgusted with yourself, lose patience, or give up if you sometimes fail to act as your philosophy dictates. But after each setback, return to reason and be content if most of your acts are worthy of a good man."

When you blend your feelings and intellect, you own a superpower. Triangulating sources you respect will help you develop it.

HERE is the rest of this essay. I call out shills, liars, and crazy people. For your purposes, they are identical. Robert Malone and Steve Kirsch are glaring examples. See Sasha Latypova's analysis HERE and Matthew Crawford's HERE.

Chapter 6
Dr. Robert Gammal's Brutal View of Dentistry, Especially Root Canals

---

I would rather have questions that can't be answered than answers that can't be questioned.

— Richard P. Feynman

LINK. Also on Rumble HERE.

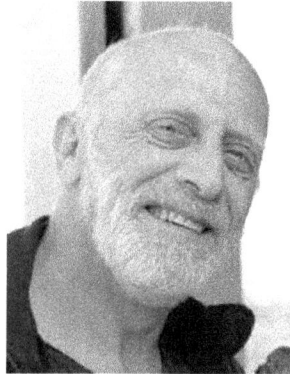

D r. Robert Gammal, an Australian dentist, coauthored this chapter. It summarizes his book *The Garbage Collector: Root Canals, Disease, and What the Dental Profession Refuses to Acknowledge* (2022). It has over 700 references and is based on Gammal's lifetime of research. It is required reading for serious students of dentistry.

Teeth consist of hard "enamel" on the outside. On the inside, there is the soft nerve and "pulp," which conducts the circulation that keeps a tooth alive. A "dentin" layer lies between these:

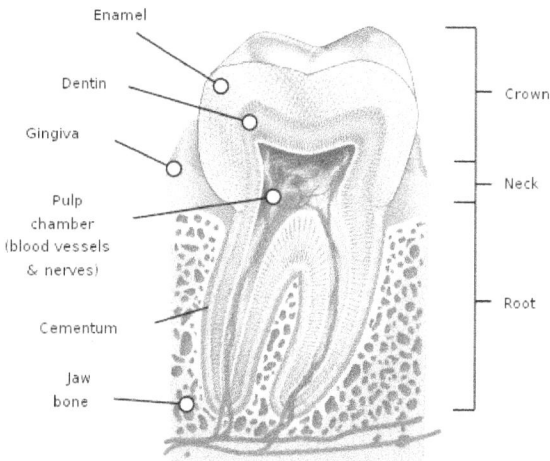

Wikipedia

Every tooth has three miles of "microtubules" that pass from the inside layers to the outside of the enamel. Bacteria and anything else in the pulp or mouth can go freely back and forth.

During a root canal procedure, the dentist drills out the tooth's center. He then applies carcinogenic antiseptics such as phenol and formaldehyde in a futile attempt to sterilize it. Next, he fills it with a range of toxic materials that are incompatible with human tissues (HERE is a list). These are all deemed safe and effective by the dental fraternity, the FDA, and the Therapeutic Goods Association of Australia. They pass freely into the brain, which is only a few centimeters away.

After a tooth is drilled out, a hole remains where the nerves passed into the root. In a vain attempt to plug this gap, mercury alloys were often used in the past. Although this is mostly out of style, other hazardous materials are still placed. But no dentist can fill it precisely, so it remains open to the rest of the body. Biological dentists remove these mummified root-canal teeth and the poisons their colleagues inserted.

Dr. Gammal writes, "All root fillings leak, and this worsens over time. The other danger is that if the root canal is overfilled with toxic filling materials, it inevitably kills the bone around the end of the root. Mercury is sometimes still placed at the end of the root following the apicectomy procedure, and this is a total disaster."

Teeth are living human tissues, not stones. Following a root canal, the tooth dies and becomes a "foreign body." All surgeons know what happens if they leave dead biological material inside a surgical wound —it becomes infected and spreads bacteria to other locations. Arthritis and other inflammatory conditions often disappear when these dead teeth—the infection source—are removed. Furthermore, nearly all heart attack artery blockages contain exactly the same types of bacteria as live in the patient's mouth.

Gammal editorializes:

Nothing works. The whole procedure is based on illusion from beginning to end. If it were possible to sterilize the tooth, then this problem would not exist. There is a blanket denial that bacteria and toxins escape from the tooth [through the microtubules] the whole way down the length of the root and not just through the apex. It would therefore make more sense to take the whole root out and not just the end of it. Fantasy and illusion reign in the minds of endodontists.

For good health, root canals must always be extracted, and the practice must be banned.

Yoho note: This introduction understates these harms, for it examines the timeline of individual root canals. What happens over the life of the patient's mouth is worse. Dentists attach bridges by carving up adjacent normal teeth. This eventually kills them and they, in turn, are drilled out into root canals. Judy's story in Chapter 1 is an example. After our kindly dentist was done with her, he had killed every tooth in her mouth but one.

If you have root canals in your mouth, study *The Garbage Collector* until you are convinced they must all be removed to preserve your health. (Note: root canals, apicectomies, and retrograde root fillings are nearly identical for our purposes.)

Dr. Gammal's heroic journey

From 1975 until 1987, Gammal placed amalgams, did root therapies, and poured fluoride over children's teeth. After this, he took three years off to study natural treatments. During this period, while he avoided personal mercury exposure, his health improved dramatically. After he returned to dentistry, Dr. Gammal studied with Dr. Hal Huggins in Colorado. He learned that reducing his patients' total body mercury by removing amalgams often produced spectacular health improvements.

Gammal says that most oral and many medical problems are caused by ill-conceived dental procedures such as tooth implants and root canals. In *The Garbage Collector*, he wrote:

When we take [this] garbage out [dead teeth and dental appliances], the body has a chance to heal. This can happen so quickly it can make your head spin.

My professors, peers, and dental association taught me to poison myself, my family, my friends, and all patients. I do not thank these people... I regard [them] at best as criminally negligent and possibly pathologically insane. The mad hatters [referring to mercury-intoxicated hat manufacturers of yesteryear] are the teachers, judges, and jurors of our great profession! These people pretend to be the guardians of dental ethics and education, and are responsible for some of the greatest suffering that mankind experiences.

Yes, I sound scathing because I am. The criminals who taught me made me responsible for creating an unknown quantity of disease. I have no idea how many people I have poisoned and killed. This is one of the greatest burdens for any dentist who takes on this new paradigm. There is no exaggeration in what I am saying. As a good, conscientious dentist, I looked after my family and friends. I did what I was told, going by what the great professors and deans taught at university. I had a chance with some of these people to undo the damage I had caused. Others died of all sorts of medical conditions caused by my "treatments." Did I really cause these deaths? Do I feel differently about the patients who are not my inner circle? No! I became a very good "sick-making" machine. I was the perfect dentist because I did everything that I was taught to do at university. Everyone suffered.

I spent the rest of my forty years in dentistry doing the opposite. In this latter period, I saw multiple sclerosis disappear after extracting one dead tooth. I saw suicide notes torn up after extracting one dead tooth. I've witnessed brain tumors disappear after extracting one dead tooth. And it goes on and on. All these dead teeth had had root canals which were done by dentists who I am sure had the best interests of their patients at heart, just as I did. The end results of their state-of-the-art treatments became glaringly obvious. The body can often heal itself very quickly if given the opportunity.

Gammal retired in 2014.

He emphasizes that the entire area around extracted teeth must be thoroughly drilled out. Contrary to customary dental practice, no part of the tooth ligament or any surrounding area that might be infected should remain. Moreover, if the underlying bony area has "cavitations," soft regions visible on the x-ray, they must also be cleaned out or infections persist. (These are sometimes more obvious on specialized three-dimensional imaging than on ordinary dental films.)

Work like this is routine for surgeons; they call it "debridement." However, the dental establishment claims it is "over-servicing." Gammal elaborates:

Many chronic degenerative diseases can be linked directly to dental treatments. Not knowing or understanding this, doctors can only treat symptoms without ever finding a cure. They, like the dentists, have been misled for far too long. They do not know that dead teeth can create cancer or that mercury may be responsible for infertility. They all believe that fluoride in drinking water stops tooth decay and that it cannot calcify your pineal gland or cause hypothyroidism, osteosarcoma, or heart disease.

Dentistry is not the only cause of chronic degenerative diseases, but it is one of the most overlooked and ignored causes. You will see later the relationships to cancers, multiple sclerosis, cardiac disease, and a vast range of other conditions.

Gammal writes about his mentors:

In 1991 I went to Colorado to study with Dr Hall Huggins. If you can get a hold of his book, It's All In Your Head, you will read the first-hand account of what follows and learn lots in the process. Dr Huggins was the man who started the third amalgam war in the 1970's, with his research into amalgam. He was the person who brought the teachings of Dr Weston Price into our current conscious-ness. He was a genius with a heart bigger than his enormous intellect. When I went to his clinic to register for the course, I was delighted by a young 8 year old girl, who was having a great time playing in the waiting room. I made comment to the receptionist about what a gorgeous happy kid she was. The receptionist said, "take a good look as she is part of your course." At the time she had come to see Dr Huggins a year earlier, she had been sent home to die, because her leukemia was untreatable.

Dr Huggins was very thorough. He had blood tests and biomarkers from the time he saw her, throughout her treatment and follow ups a month, 6 months and a year later. What was the treatment? Dr Huggins removed a tooth that had been 'treated' with a pulpotomy and covered with a stainless steel crown. The pulpotomy was performed about a year earlier and she was diagnosed with leukemia a month after the dental treatment. Within a week of this tooth being removed, her white cell count returned to normal. A month later she was told that the leukemia had disappeared. One year later there was still no trace of cancer.

In the latter half of my dental career, I was exposed to the teachings of people like Dr Hal Huggins, Dr Horst Poehlman, Prof Boyd Haley, Prof Murray Vimy, Prof Vera Stejskal, Dr Jerry Bouquot and in the written word, Dr Weston Price, to name but a few of the great thinkers with the courage to talk about their knowledge. They patiently taught me as I violently rejected their claims.

This is when I learnt about the true cost of leaving dead teeth in the mouth. This is when I started to learn that the forced medication, called water fluoridation, had no beneficial effects at all. This is when I learnt that the mercury I was implanting into patient's bodies was causing mercury poisoning, with all the horrifying ramifications that this entails. I learnt that by using mercury amalgam as a filling material, I was also poisoning myself and my staff. There was at last a reason for the uncontrollable trembling hands, muscle twitches and splitting headaches, as well an explanation of the acute optic neuritis and rapid mood swings.

Dr Huggins was once asked if all root-canalled teeth should be removed. He replied that it was only "for those people who had an interest in their health."

Dr. Gammal discusses why root canal procedures invariably fail:

Not one of the god-endodontists has a way of measuring the sterility of the tooth. In fact, there is no measure of sterility at all. It is impossible to sterilize the canal, so there is not really any standard by which we can judge whether the tooth is ready to be filled. Because they had to admit failure regarding their ability to sterilize teeth, they created a new term. They now claim to be able to take the teeth to a state of "physiologic balance." There is no such thing as physiologic balance!

When the tooth is ready to be filled is a guess based on a lack of pain and 'no stinky smell'. The decision to fill the canal and finish the treatment is based only on the dentist's appraisal of how much he or she can get away with. Spending too much time on such a tooth erodes the profit margin. It is neither a scientific nor a logical decision. All root-canalled teeth are infected. The bone around all of these teeth is infected.

All materials used in the root canal procedure are toxic. Some will affect the nervous system. Some will affect a developing foetus. Some will cause cancer. There is not one which is biocompatible. All these materials will escape from the tooth and spread around the whole of your body. They can cause all sorts of diseases in any part of your body.

German physician and cancer specialist Professor Max Daunderer is contemptuous of dentistry. Gammal quotes a 1998 interview with him:

The dental work we get from dentists is not something biological or medical. I'd say it is a technical thing, and the techniques give the dentists a number of very strong poisons to be implanted in the mouth. If you kill the tooth and then fill its root canal with mercury, formalde-

hyde, cortisodentistry is just a sin against the biology of the body and a sin against the 'real' medicine.

Dr. Gammal says titanium implants are also failures:

These good-looking X-rays of dead teeth do not show the infection around or in the roots. No matter how good the tooth looks on an X-ray, it will still be infected.

For the bone surrounding the implant to become infected from this source, the bacteria have to have "escaped" from the dead tooth and penetrated the bone. If they are in the bone, then they will be carried everywhere else in the body. If these bugs decide that your heart is a good home, then you might just have a heart attack. They might decide to inhabit your brain instead and create neurological cancers or MS. They might localize in your ears and cause deafness.

All bacteria and the toxins they produce can and do travel out of the tooth to the rest of your body. It is not just the implant that might fail in this case. In any language, this is a focal infection arising from the source.

Titanium implants are alloy blends. Each of these metals can potentially cause toxicity, or worse, allergy. Some manufacturers consider their products' contents trade secrets, which impedes diagnosis of metal allergies. Also, electrical currents between implants, tooth fillings, and orthopedic appliances routinely create issues such as toxic metal shedding. All these issues result in chronic inflammation and infection.

To avoid these problems, ceramic (zirconia) has been recently used for implant manufacture. Since these are not metal, they are nearly biologically inert. Surgeons implanting them must have the skills to remove all areas of mouth infection, bone graft, and implant the artificial teeth during a single surgery. Stem cells and ozone should also be used. This may take half a day. If these precautions are not followed, chronic infections ensue.

As of late 2023, pricing for these seems predatory. For example, one patient in California was charged $200,000 for four implants. Costs are more reasonable in other countries.

Gammal about mercury and root canals:

Dentistry does not consider mercury from amalgam to be a problem, either. Mercury is the third most toxic element known to science. Arsenic is the "first" most toxic. Lead is somewhere in between. There is no amount of mercury that is safe. None. The manufacturer states that this material causes cancer. Why in the name of sanity does a health care profession want to implant it into living bodies? Why do the TGA and FDA give approval for its use, especially in children?

Hundreds of studies prove that root canals destroy health:

Just one short list published in the International Endodontic Journal, titled "Root canal treatment and general health: a review of the literature," is testimony to this: "There has been an increase in the number of case reports published in the medical literature citing dental infection as an associated factor in several systemic illnesses including; • uveitis (Sela & Sharav 1979) (inflammation of the middle layer of tissue in the eye) • intracranial abscess (Holin et al. 1967, Henig et al. 1978, Ingham et al. 1978, Churton & Green 1980, Aldous et al. 1987, Marks et al. 1988, Saal et al. 1988) (brain abscess) • childhood hemiplegia (Hamlyn 1978), cerebral infarction (Syrjanen et al. 1989), acteriospermia and subfertility (Bieniek & Riedel 1993) (brain damage or spinal cord injury that leads to paralysis on one side of the body) necrotizing fasciitis (Gallia & Johnson 1981, Steel 1987, Stoykewych et al. 1978) (a bacterial infection that results in the death of parts of the body's soft tissue. It is a severe disease of sudden onset that spreads rapidly.) • mediastinitis (Hendler & Quinn 1978, Zachariades et al. 1988, Musgrove & Malden 1989) (inflammation or infection of the mediastinum) • fatal endocarditis (Kralovic et al. 1995) (infection of the lining of the heart) • toxic shock syndrome

(Egbert et al. 1987, Navazesh et al. 1994) (acute septicaemia typically caused by bacterial infection) Septicaemia (Lee 1984) (Bacterial Blood Poisoning)

A small taste of the current literature shows that dead teeth can cause a wide range of diseases: • immune system diseases • infection of hip replacements • abscess of eyes • cervical cellulites and mediastenitis • Necrotizing fascitis • coronary atherosclerosis • sinusitis • Multiple Sclerosis • brain abscess • brain cancer • central nervous system damage • Trigeminal Neuralgia

Infection spreading from teeth may cause the following: • Osteomyelitis of the mandible • Maxillary sinusitis and orbital abscess • Wound botulism • Ludwig's angina (Heart) • Necrotizing fasciitis • Cavernous sinus thrombosis (brain) Persistent pyrexia of unknown origin (high temperature) • Septicaemia—Streptococcus milleri and Pseudomonas Septicaemia with disseminated intravascular coagulation • Pulmonary abscess (lung) • Pyogenic hepatic abscess (liver) • Brain abscess • Brain abscess and acute meningitis • Paraspinal abscess and paraplegia (spine) • Bacterial endocarditis (heart) • Splenic abscess (spleen) • Mediastinal abscess and pneumonia (chest)

The following diseases are listed in a paper entitled "Systemic Diseases Caused By Oral Infection", published in 2000: "Cardiovascular disease, coronary heart disease: atherosclerosis and myocardial infarction, stroke, infective endocarditis, bacterial pneumonia, low birth weight & diabetes mellitus, cerebral infarction, acute myocardial infarction, abnormal pregnancy outcome, persistent pyrexia, idiopathic trigeminal neuralgia, toxic shock syndrome, systemic granulocytic cell defects, chronic meningitis." (Published in Microbiology Reviews - This paper has 158 references) The bacteria in a tooth can and do travel throughout the body. There is now research which demonstrates the presence of oral bacteria in the uterus and amniotic fluid. These uterine infections can lead to preterm birth in pregnant women.

Dr. Gammal concludes:

Research about the dangers of mercury from amalgam fillings has been around since its inception in 1812. Research about the dangers of root canal procedures has been around since the early 1920's. Research about the dangers of fluoride has been around for over 80 years. There is no reason to suggest it does not exist, especially when the current research fully supports the older research.

The amount of mercury in the mouth of a person with fillings was on average 2.5 grams, enough to contaminate five ten-acre lakes to the extent there would be dangerous levels in fish. (Electric Power Research Institute, EPRI Technical Brief. "Mercury in the Environment", 1993; & EPRI Journal, April 1990.)

Dr. Gammal told dozens of stunning stories about patients cured after removing their metals and rotten, infected teeth.

[While] I was hopeful that taking out the dead teeth would help, I was shocked to see the speed at which the body can heal when the rubbish is removed. It was terrifying to see my patients come back a week later to have the stitches removed and report that the symptoms they had suffered with, sometimes for years, had disappeared within a matter of days.

One of the most common stories that I heard was that of breast lumps. I lost count of the number of women who told me their breast lumps had disappeared after a root-canalled tooth was removed. This often happened within a week of the tooth coming out. The psychological stress of living with lumps in the breast is one thing. The very real rise in the incidence of breast cancer is another.

Arthritis is [frequently] associated with dead teeth. A relevant case study appears in the 2002 literature. This report describes a remission of rheumatoid arthritis (RA) of 16 years duration, apparently caused by the extraction of endodontically well-treated, healthy looking teeth. The only clue that the teeth were contributing to the disease pathogenesis in this case of RA was that the patient was able to reproducibly induce severe attacks of arthritis after prolonged, heavy pressure on

some of his teeth treated with root canal fillings. After extraction, a
small pus layer was found to cover the apices of the clinically healthy-
looking teeth. The rheumatoid factor (RF) became negative and the
patient remained symptom free for the next 16 years.

Multiple Sclerosis (MS) cures:

Quoting Professor Daunderer, "if we take Multiple Sclerosis
patients who removed amalgam but refused both extraction of root
canals and treatment of infected maxillary bone, we observe a cure
rate from MS of 16%. But when we consider multiple sclerosis
patients that beside amalgam removal accepted our full treatment
(root canal extraction and cleaning of alveolar bone), the percentage of
cures increases to 86."

In the 1970s and 1980s, Professor Patrick Stortebecker, who was
then the Professor of Neural Surgery at the Karolinska Institute in
Sweden, demonstrated that the primary lesion in Multiple Sclerosis is
not demyelenation but instead is an infected plaque around the venous
side of the blood supply to the brain. Cerebral MS plaques showed the
same organisms as found in dead teeth, periodontal disease, and other
oral infections. Spinal MS lesions showed the same organisms that are
found in the bowel and vagina.

Stortebecker described the pathway of transmission through the
non-valved venous plexus for both areas. By injecting dyes into the
angle of the mandible (therefore not a bony connection to the rest of the
skull), he was able to fill the whole of the intra-cranial blood vessels.
This demonstrated that the non-valved veinous plexus below the skull
allows movement of blood in both directions. This is critical to the
understanding of how the microorganisms from the mouth could enter
the brain.

Causal comparison of the WHO map of dental caries incidences
throughout the world reveals a striking parallel in general trend.
Comparison of decayed, missing and filled teeth with the MS death
rates results in a correlation coefficient of 0.97, and the probability of a
chance occurrence is less than 0.002. This represents a nearly perfect
linear relationship between dental disease rates and MS death rates.

From the work of Professor Vera Stejskal in Europe, it is clear that all metals must be avoided in Multiple Sclerosis patients. This includes the metals in composite resins that are used to colour the filling materials. Porcelains should be the filling material of choice and should be cemented into place with old-fashioned but safer zinc phosphate cement. For all those with an autoimmune disease, I strongly recommend you read the information at www.melisa.org.

MS patient stories:

Bill was another patient who came to see me in desperation because, at the age of thirty-two, he figured that he was too young for an MS diagnosis. The treatment he received was the removal of a single root-canalled tooth. Of course, our surgical procedure involved removing the periodontal ligament and unhealthy bone from the cavity. Bill stated the following: In September 2003, I went along to my dentist and had a root canal treatment performed. Months later in January 2004, I started to experience problems with my balance, tingling sensations and numbness in my hands and feet. Subsequently I was referred to a neurologist and after many tests – C.T. scans, lumbar puncture etc, – I was told that the probable cause of my problems was Multiple Sclerosis. The amazing thing for me was I had this root canal filled tooth pulled out in September 2004 and a week later, literally a week later, my balance started to improve, and the sensations that I had been experiencing for 9 months, started to abate. The numbness & tingling – and basically things have just improved from there. It is now December 2005!633

A lady in her forties—Helen, for want of a name—came to see me after being diagnosed with MS. She had a few young children and a great relationship with her husband. She was very happy but felt that she was too young to be sent home with a death sentence and no hope of treatment. On examining her mouth, I found one root-canalled tooth on the upper left and a small metal-and-porcelain bridge to replace a missing front tooth. There wasn't any amalgam in her mouth.

Technically, the bridge was very well made, but we had no idea which metals were used. The root canal looked like a job that any endodontist would be proud of, and there was no abscess visible on the X-ray. No matter what the tooth looks like on an X-ray, all dead teeth remain infected, as it is impossible to sterilize them. She'd had great mechanical dentistry done. She also brought in her MRI scan, which showed two large lesions in her brain.

She had done her research and requested that I take out the bridge and the dead tooth. I told her there was no promise it would affect her health, as I always did, and she accepted this completely. I also agreed with her that there was a good likelihood the MS could be related to these. At this first appointment, she decided to remove both the tooth and the bridge immediately. She was not interested in proving which was a cause. She just wanted to eliminate all possible causes.

She was quite happy to go home with a "gappy" smile. Three months later, Helen came back in to see me with a new MRI. All of her symptoms had resolved, and the MRI scan was clear of any lesions. Her neurologist had declared her free of MS and did not want to know what she had done to make such a radical change.

The symptoms of mercury poisoning and those of multiple sclerosis are identical. The main source of mercury to the general population is, of course, dental amalgam. In fact, mercury exposure occurs at a rate ten times higher through this source than through all other sources combined, including seafood. 634 Studies have found mercury-related mental effects to be indistinguishable from those of MS.

Many MS patients have been helped by reducing their mercury loads. This can be achieved only if the source of the mercury is removed. Thus, all amalgam fillings need to go, as well as all other sources of mercury, including amalgam tattoos. Several published studies have clearly demonstrated an improvement of symptoms after the amalgams are removed. Not all recover, but many do. Amalgam may be an important risk factor for patients with autoimmune diseases.

Dr Huggins noted that the incidence of both ALS and MS started *going through the roof after 1976, with the introduction of high-copper amalgams, which release about fifty times more mercury than the older formulations of amalgam with less copper. Multiple Sclerosis was not known before 1830, when mercury amalgam became a worldwide phenomenon!*

Dr. Gammal saw hundreds of tumors disappear three to four months after he removed root canal teeth. Here are opinions from oncologists who understand this:

Dr Issels, Daunderer, and many others have rated their treatments as only average, unless the dental work is done first. Then their success rates increased to about 80 percent. This is a far cry from the miserable cure rates of chemotherapy and radiotherapy. According to a 2004 report by Morgan, Ward, and Barton, "The contribution of cytotoxic chemotherapy to 5-year survival in adult malignancies ... survival in adults was estimated to be 2.3% in Australia and 2.1% in the USA." 578

Dr Issels found that 98 percent of his cancer patients had between two and ten dead teeth.

Try looking up the success rate of radiation therapy, and you will find a never-ending array of articles claiming a 95 percent success rate for Prostate Cancer ONLY. No other type of cancer is mentioned. Also, no mention is made that radiation is itself carcinogenic. The use of radiation started as a bad experiment in the 1920s but proved to be too profitable to discard.

Gammal writes:

Most of the degenerative diseases of our times are regarded as having "no known causes." Potential causes are linked to genetic and environmental conditions when you ask the doctor the why, what, and how. Many of these diseases have "societies" attached to them for the support of patients and research. For as long as I can remember, the evening news has carried regular stories of trial treatments for cancer, which are always in their research stage. The level of depression in our society has gone through the roof. Behavioral problems in children are also increasing at alarming rates. There seems to be a potential vaccine for just about any disease, even including those that are not infectious like the human papilloma viruses that cause cervical cancer.

When there's no known cause, there can never be a cure. Gradually the "no known cause" becomes a part of the language and the thinking of both doctor and patient. There is an acceptance amongst most people that if there is 'no known cause', then it is just bad luck. Perhaps it is your genetic makeup? The genetic argument never states as much but strongly implies that if you have a particular genetic weakness in some area, then that's what's going to kill you. We all have genetic weaknesses, as well as genetic strengths. To a point, this totally explains the variety of diseases found by both Price and Rosenow. Many of these conditions may not kill you but will certainly reduce your quality of life.581 Perhaps it is time to look in other directions for a cause.

He concludes:

There is now more than sufficient published research that demonstrates the role of oral infections as a cause of heart disease, diabetes, kidney disease, multiple sclerosis, and other neurological diseases to call for an immediate ban on the practice of keeping dead teeth in the body. It is time for the dental profession to take responsibility for the disasters they cause.

Like Watergate, the most criminal part of this story is the coverup. Dentists who know the truth are pressured to keep their mouths shut. If they advertise or even mention to patients that removing amalgams or root canals improves health, their state boards may censor or revoke their licenses.

References

Root Cause (2018) is a documentary about cancer and heart attacks and their relation to dead teeth. Interviews include one of America's leading cardiologists, Dr Thomas Levy, who made it clear that infection from root canals causes heart disease. Every root canal is infected and stays infected. You can buy or rent this movie or search for a free version.

Dr. Gammal's website realdentalinfo.com is HERE. He describes the care that must be taken to avoid poisoning the patient when removing mercury.

Dr. Gammal tells us how to evaluate dentists HERE. If possible, find one trained by the International Academy of Oral Medicine and Toxicology (IAOMT).

Dr. Gammal's fluoride presentation. This is a free download for anyone to use.

Quecksilber is Gammal's 2004 documentary about the dangers of mercury from dental amalgam. More recently, he produced *Rooted*, a movie about the dangers of root canals.

The Roots of Disease and The Toxic Tooth by Robert Kulacz and Thomas Levy

Curing the Incurable by Thomas Levy.

Solving The M.S. Mystery: Help, Hope and Recovery by Dr Hal Huggins. Order it HERE.

Dr. David Minkoff's excellent interview on YouTube about root canals.

Cancer: A Second Opinion by Dr Issels. He devotes a chapter to dental causes.

Parting shots

From Dr. Gammal's book:

The hatters of old used to cure rabbit fur with mercuric nitrate. They had profound psychiatric manifestations—they went quite bonkers. They became as "mad as a hatter", as clearly demonstrated in Alice's Adventures in Wonderland! Many patients who have amalgam implanted into their mouths also become mad from the mercury they're exposed to. Any dentist who uses or drills out amalgam will also be mercury poisoned and often will also become as mad as a hatter. Should we wonder why dentists have the highest suicide rate of all professions?

Adolf Hitler... refused to listen to his generals' advice to quit whilst ahead. WW2 could have ended in 1943, but Hitler had numerous amalgams, along with two gold bridges and crowns, which would have guaranteed a continuous flood of mercury to his [brain.]

Fluoride in the drinking water also has profound psychological effects. Fluoride will lower IQs across a whole population. 646,647 It was put in drinking water in German concentration camps to keep the inmates more apathetic. It is used in our water supply for the same reason. Both mercury and fluoride act as inhibitors of brain growth and maturity when foetuses are exposed in utero. Neither is in any way beneficial...

A forty-six-year-old male restaurant owner... for many years suffered with chronic fungal infections in and around his fingernails. He had, like most of the patients I see, tried everything to get rid of this, as it had a profound effect on his ability to work with food. Within one month of removing a dead tooth and doing some periodontal cleaning, all of the troublesome infections had gone. In his words: "it is now time that I should say that I am breathing a lot easier. I can breathe in without opening my mouth all day long. The same at night – I can breathe in without breathing through my mouth. Whereas before was completely the opposite ..." He told me his story while showing me how he could use his fingers as drumsticks on the table. This was impossible before because of the excruciating pain.

From *Kiss Your Dentist Goodbye: A Do-It-Yourself Mouth Care System for Healthy, Clean Gums and Teeth* (2017) by Ellie Phillips, DDS:

Almost all American adults have damage from dental disease as they age, and almost a quarter of all adults between sixty-five and seventy-four have severe disease. In the United States today, around 30 percent of adults age sixty-five have no teeth at all. Many people, despite visits to their dentist, are never cured of their disease, but they continue to require treatments year after year, with repairs becoming constantly more extensive. Dental visits are often a maintenance system that does not stop the disease but, rather, simply keeps the symptoms within limits that you, the consumer, agree to accept. Patients have been conditioned to view fillings and repairs as normal, as problems that are part of the aging process, and their ongoing dental treatments as something they deserve.

Dr. Phillips believes xylitol non-nutritive sweeteners promote tooth health.

Chapter 7
Ezekiel Lagos, DDS, Operates in a Hazmat Suit to Save Patient Lives

My excellent adventure in Tijuana

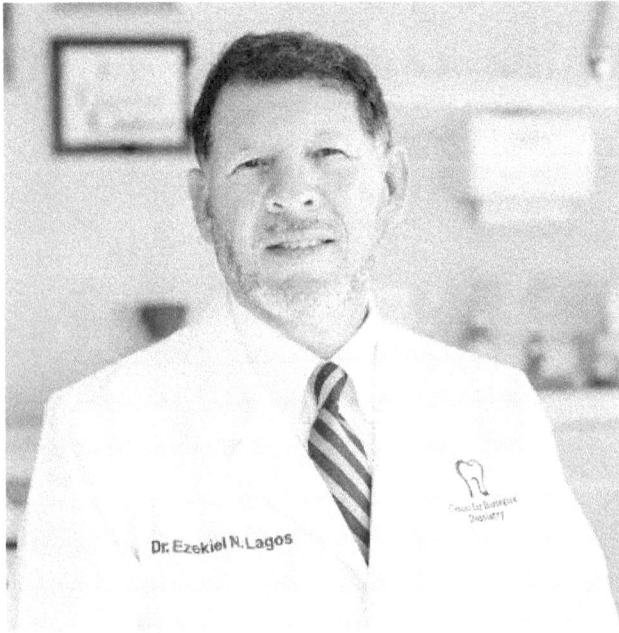

LINK

In May 2023, I knew nothing about dentists, the toxic substances they use, or the chronic, health-damaging infections they cause. I started researching because I learned that the mercury in my fillings might be causing my tremors. I began by reading *Toxic Teeth: How a Biological (Holistic) Dentist Can Help You Cure Cancer, Facial Pain, Autoimmune, Heart, and Other Disease Caused By Infected Gums, Root Canals, Jawbone Cavitations, and Toxic Metals* by J.M. Swartz M.D. et al. (2019).

I was horrified by Swartz's portrayal of dentistry, so when I visited my Los Angeles dentist for tooth cleaning a few weeks later, I asked him how many mercury amalgams I had. After clicking on my teeth, he replied, "Seventeen." I nearly fell out of the chair.

Dr. Swartz had been Dr. Lagos's patient and recommended him in his book, so I sent Dr. Lagos my "panorex" mouth X-ray. He was so busy that he could not see me until mid-August.

As I continued studying, my paranoia meter started flashing red. I realized that just stepping into a dental office is hazardous. The dentist in the next room might be drilling without the protections used by biological dentists. Even if I was only there for tooth cleaning, I might inhale mercury and other poisons.

My health was not my only concern. I soon learned that out-of-control dentistry operating for profit is responsible for a double-digit percentage of all US health problems. Not only are people suffering, but the unsustainable costs are borne by all of us.

During this period, I saw a neurologist about my tremor. She immediately told me I had Parkinson's disease (PD). Since this is the second most common disease her specialty sees after Alzheimer's (AD), it was obvious to her.

She asked me if I had started falling yet (not yet!). It reminded me of a time when I used an ammunition storage bag as an airplane carry-on and mistakenly left a couple of shotgun shells in a zippered pocket. The security asked me if I had been arrested yet (not yet!).

Neurologists diagnose conditions, but Pharma dictates their treatments. I asked her about the holistic remedies I wrote about in a recent post, and she said firmly, "None of it works." She must have felt bad about it, so she apologized for the delay in her appointment. I replied, "Absolutely, no worries." From my research, I already knew that our modern "Rockefeller Medicine*" generally only treated symptoms. They offered no cures or anything that even slowed the progress of PD. I was on my own.

*Rockefeller commissioned the Flener Report in 1910. It purportedly recommended better medical science, but had many adverse effects, including boosting corporate control of doctors.

I increased the pace of my already manic research. I learned that pesticides, electromagnetic fields (EMFs), and certain metals, including mercury, are linked to several brain degeneration syndromes. These include Parkinson's, Alzheimer's, autism, and amyotrophic lateral sclerosis (ALS). These are dubbed "idiopathic." This means that their causes are mysterious and even unknowable. Since Pharma makes no money on cures or inexpensive treatments, they ignore or disparage them.

My functional doctor friends told me to get my mercury amalgams removed first. Although Swartz was a strong referral source, I evaluated Dr. Lagos carefully. I knew that I had little recourse if I had problems in Mexico.

Dr. Lagos was trained by Hal Huggins, DDS, the grandfather of the holistic dental movement. He pioneered biological dentistry and spoke against mercury fillings and other dangerous procedures.

I am a seasoned observer of doctors and medical offices, for I trained to be a surgical center inspector and have visited hundreds of facilities. Lagos's website, reviews, credentials, and office documents were top-notch. My experience with him later confirmed these impressions. I found the following on his wall of diplomas:

The Multi-Disciplined Alliance

"First Do No Harm"

The Multi-Disciplined Alliance was created by Dr. Hal A. Huggins to give patients desiring his *Protocol* a better opportunity to receive what they expect. The "Alliance" is composed of professionals that will commit to performing certain levels of competence in the effort to "FIRST DO NO HARM".

*D*r. Huggins and his team train the "Alliance" dentists and their staff in the use of programs to practice the protocol of safety and recovery. The "Alliance" member provides a safe environment for patients desiring to rid themselves of amalgam fillings and dental materials. They can also assist their patients in obtaining the proper detoxification, chelating and recovery programs that are aligned with the protocol.

*I*n 1979, Dr. Huggins found that improper amalgam removal can cause the onset of autoimmune diseases *that were not there previously*, so over the years he has developed a *Protocol* that potentially provides far more benefit than risk for the patient. A survey of patients who had called Dr. Huggins office over a two year period for a referral dentist provided the following statistical result: Of the patients who had dental treatment performed, the ones who went to an "Alliance" dentist reported no illness or ill effects after their revision. For those who went to a non-Alliance dentist, sixty-three percent (63%) reported that they had contracted or suffered from a disease or ailment, that they had not had previous to dental treatment, directly following their dental revision.

*M*ore recently, Dr. Huggins has found through clinical research and observation that root canals pose a serious threat to patient health. It took years to bring the amalgam issue to the forefront, but that will not be the case regarding the dangers of root canal toxins. Again, the "Alliance" dentist is well educated and prepared to safely provide the necessary alternatives and corrective actions involved in dealing with root canals, cavitations and other toxins.

*F*inally, the "Alliance" has provided the opportunity for these dedicated professionals to consult directly with Dr. Huggins in order to insure that the most demanding situations will be handled confidently. Another great benefit of the "Alliance" is the ability to network, confer and to exchange ideas with other members in order to further promote their commitment to provide the highest level of excellence in service to their patients.

Who Does The "Alliance" Benefit?

Patients and professionals who desire non-toxic dental materials and procedures as well as a proven potential for recovery.

Lagos is a member of the International Academy of Oral Medicine and Toxicology (IAOMT) and a Huggins Alliance Member. Dr. Lagos recommended that I have Biocomp laboratories blood tests to see if I was sensitive to dental materials. It showed that I was reacting to several metals, including mercury and aluminum.

I was at his office for five days. For the first four, I had intravenous sedation up to six hours a day. It was tolerable but not my idea of a great time. I had no pain during or after surgery except for a few days of aches after my dead wisdom tooth removal on the last day.

Here is what the procedure looked like; that is me under there. I am wearing nasal oxygen. A space blanket over me keeps me warm and provides full-body protection during amalgam removal. I received 50 grams of intravenous vitamin C each day.

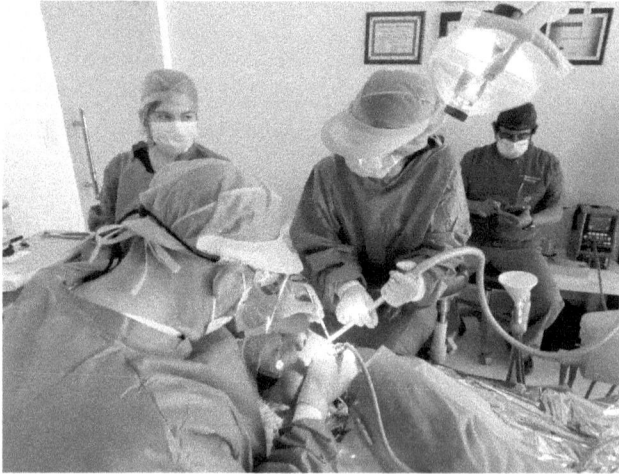

The anesthesiologist is checking his stocks, but they do that everywhere.

Los Angeles dentists sometimes charge thousands to fix a single tooth. My total fees were less than $7000. The five-star Quartz Hotel near the clinic cost me $150 a night.

Three weeks later, my tremors and tinnitus were a little better. I was salivating excessively, however, which was a new Parkinson's symptom. A bit of mercury exposure during the removals was inevitable.

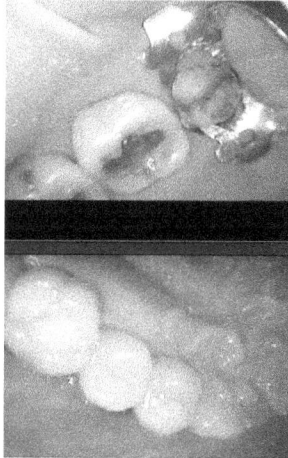

Samples of my before/after photos.

EDTA (Ethylenediaminetetraacetic acid) chelation is the traditional approach to heavy metal removal, but my research indicates it is a mistake. After initially binding the mercury, EDTA drops it, and it redistributes to the rest of the body. This can damage the kidneys. The safer and more effective approach is intravenous phosphatidylcholine. See Chapter 11.

Dr. Lagos' office documents (available in ebook)

My treatment schedule. Download
"Jonas's Guide to Dr Lagos." Download
Patient And Caregiver Information. Download

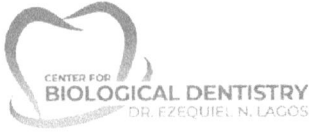

CENTER FOR BIOLOGICAL DENTISTRY

(619) 879-3131
www.biologicaldent.com

Ave. Paseo del Centenario 9580,
Suite 2102,
Zona Urbana Rio, Tijuana, Mexico

Books by Dr. Huggins:

It's All In Your Head: The Link Between Mercury Amalgams and Illness

    Uninformed Consent: The Hidden Dangers in Dental Care
    It's All in Your Head: Diseases Caused by Silver-Mercury Fillings
    Who Makes Your Hormones Hum???
    Solving the MS Mystery: Help, Hope and Recovery

Other sources:

Biocom Labs, founded by the late Dr. Hal Huggins, is the lab Lagos recommends for biocompatibility testing of dental materials. They accept blood samples by mail. DNA Connexions is their sister laboratory.

Quicksilver Scientific is a detox program. They send you the supplements you need for detoxification and also offer courses to health professionals. (I have no experience with them.)

Oasis of Hope Hospital offers alternative medicine. The late Dr. Ernesto Contreras was the founder, and he pioneered alternative medicine in Tijuana. His son, Dr. Francisco Contreras, is now in charge, and the administrator is Eduardo Ruiz. If you have cancer or another serious diagnosis, you should look at them and others. The Quartz Hotel will give you a free ride to and from this hospital.

Notes

Crossing the border can be a hassle, but Dr. Lagos's drivers make it easy. They pick you up at the San Diego airport or train station and take you to your hotel for $80.

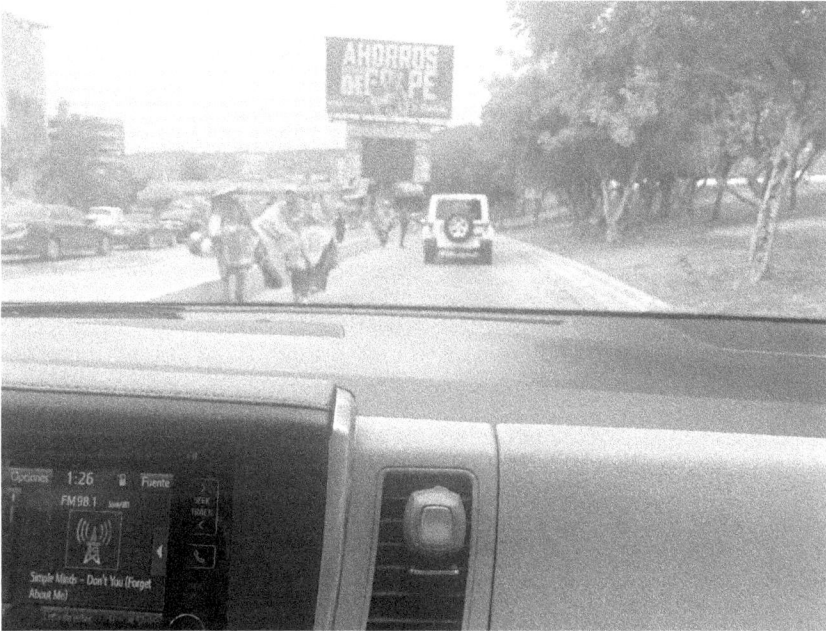

Crossing back into California from Tijuana.

I knew I should ask for nonmetallic materials, and my advisers recommended Saremco ceramic composite fillings. Lagos said, "I use Admira, which is highly biocompatible and on the list the lab gave us of your least-reactive materials."

Dr. Lagos recommends oil pulling for oral care.

Like Dr. Huggins, Lagos recommends waiting a month after amalgam removal before starting a detox.

I saw post-operative hair transplant patients at my hotel. Since I performed this procedure while practicing, I could tell their surgeon was skilled. They said they paid only 50 cents per graft.

Chapter 8
Fluoride is Devastating

Study hard what interests you the most in the most undisciplined, irreverent, and original manner possible.

— Richard P. Feynman, Nobel Prize-winning physicist

LINK

Y*oho note: I used the following sources because they offered clarity or authority. No quoted author is responsible for the following because I abridged their work and may have inadvertently changed their emphasis.*

Steve Kirsch's fluoride outline

Jay Sanders of fluoridealert.org approached me at an event and asked, "Can I give you a book?" It was the sort of life-changing question that got Robert F. Kennedy Jr. to realize that vaccines aren't safe. He gave me a copy of *The Case Against Fluoride: How Hazardous Waste Ended Up in Our Drinking Water and the Bad Science and Powerful Politics That Keep It There* (2010) by Paul Connett, James Beck, and H. Spedding Micklem.

Studies began in 1945, and fluoridation was approved in 1950 before any trials were completed or any comprehensive studies were published. Proponents claimed a tiny benefit for fluoride if it is kept in your mouth and not swallowed. Once you swallow, the risks strongly outweigh the benefits. Along with other adverse effects, children's IQs drop significantly if their mothers are exposed during pregnancy.

All large towns in California are required to fluoridate (CA Law AB733). Although no federal fluoridation law exists, almost all large U.S. cities are fluoridated. The ADA is an extremely powerful lobby. (*Yoho comment: When you finish this book, you will know who controls the ADA.*)

Short-term ways to avoid fluoride include drinking fresh or bottled spring water or distilled water. Reverse osmosis filters also work, and Culligan's is popular. Less recommended are Berkey fluoride filters. They require frequent replacement and must be kept from drying out, which makes them maintenance-intensive. There are some controversies about this filter. Another brand, the 3-stage Clearly Filtered system, rapidly loses its ability to filter fluoride after the first few fills.

To change fluoridation policies, work to get your town and state to outlaw fluoridation and donate to fluoridealert.org. Like vaccines, the science is established, but nobody wants to look at it.

Comment by the anonymous "A Midwestern Doctor"

I have been studying fluoride for a long time and have only drunk reverse osmosis (RO) water since I first learned about it as a teenager. Here are a few main points:

✪ Fluoride is difficult to filter from water; RO is one of the only reliable approaches. If you do that, you must supplement your diet with magnesium. If you use spring water, you must pick a brand with little fluoride.

✪ Many industries, notably aluminum and phosphate refiners, produce fluoride as a byproduct of their process. These industries ran into repeated issues with poisoning or killing workers in the surrounding communities when they had fluoride gas leaks. Hence, the industry concocted the idea of saying fluoride was good for teeth to get them out of lawsuit liability (it could be argued in court that fluoride cannot be toxic if it is good for teeth). Despite heavy pressure, the FDA was unwilling to grant them this due to the evidence of harm and absence of benefit from fluoride.

✪ When the Manhattan Project was being conducted, uranium centrifuges did not yet exist, so the only way to enrich uranium for nuclear weapons was to dissolve it in fluoride and separate the resulting gases by density. Based on national security, it was decided that fluoride needed to go into the water so that we could make atomic weapons and win the war. Bill Clinton declassified documents describing this (see *The Fluoride Deception,* 2006).

✪ The best book I have seen that explains the pathologic effects of fluoride is *Fluoride the Aging Factor* (1993) by John Yiamouyiannis. He makes the case that fluoride, at a very low dose, disrupts the structures of many proteins in the body due to its high electronegativity, interfering with the hydrogen bonds they depend on for their three-dimensional stability. The most common side effect observed is the weakening of collagen in the body. In areas where individuals have high amounts of fluoride in their water (a few villages in India were the best examples), they age quickly and have a weakened or deformed bone structure. Having looked at this for a while, I believe that fluoride does long-term damage to bones (this may also come from fluoride chemically altering the bones, which, in theory, is how it "helps" your teeth).

✪ Water fluoridation significantly increases cancer rates (*Fluoride the Aging Factor*).

✪ Fluoride causes adverse endocrine effects. The primary one is that it weakens the thyroid gland. Hypothyroidism is now prevalent, and it is one of the most frequent issues that integrative medicine practitioners treat and sometimes achieve miraculous results with. One, but not the only, potential cause is fluoride exposure. This is likely due to the thyroid gland substituting the iodine it needs with fluoride from water sources. A related issue is bromide. Until about twenty years ago, flour and bread were fortified with the critical nutrient iodine. Bromide has been substituted. (Hyperthyroidism was previously treated by bathing in fluoridated water.)

✪ The most concerning effects of fluoride are neuropsychiatric. The magnitude is difficult to quantify; some think that the amounts we are exposed to in the water are sufficient to cause brain effects, but others believe higher doses, such as those received from fluorinated pharmaceuticals, are necessary. One story that has gone around for a long time is that the Nazis fluorinated the water of the Jewish ghettos to make them more submissive and compliant. I tried to find a primary source for this, and I went as far back as someone in the US military saying it was done, but I never found direct verification. I have seen those effects in individuals who have taken fluorinated pharmaceuticals, particularly antidepressants.

✪ Many of the drugs with the highest rates of adverse events have fluoride structures. I always look at the chemical structure of a pharmaceutical before I consider prescribing it.

The most common fluorinated medicines that cause significant problems are fluoroquinolone antibiotics such as Cipro and fluorinated SSRI antidepressants such as Prozac. The dose you get from medications such as these over the long term is much higher than what you might be exposed to in water.

Some antifungals, such as fluconazole, the cheapest one on the market, are fluoridated. It causes reactions in some people who take it for mold issues. The others that are not fluoridated are much more expensive and typically not covered by insurance.

✪ There is no evidence that fluoride has benefits, and many have been fighting for decades to get it out of the water supply (with a few successes in recent years!). Some forms of fluoride are much more toxic than others, and typically, the more toxic industrial fluoride waste products are what end up in the water supply rather than sodium fluoride, which is still dangerous enough that it can hospitalize children who swallow too much toothpaste.

✪ Many believe fluoride disrupts mitochondrial function. When I last looked into this, there was a case for it, but there was no solid proof.

✪ Various relatively simple measures dramatically help dental health but are rarely considered. However, since dentists believe fluoridation is the solution to everything, they prescribe high-fluoride toothpaste instead.

✪ Studies have shown that drinking fluoridated water lowers IQ. This could either be due to hypothyroidism or a direct effect on the brain. Sadly, many infant formulas are advertised as being fluorinated.

✪ I am immensely frustrated by public health. Their efforts are directed at giving as many vaccinations as possible and fluorinating as many water supplies as possible. They are unenthusiastic about other policies.

✪ Public health "professionals" never consider that people have individual reactions to different drugs and doses. Some tolerate medications poorly, even at tiny doses. This is one reason among many that no medical intervention should ever be indiscriminately administered through the water supply.

Yoho comments:

About 25 percent of prescription drugs contain fluoride. These include:

✪ Statins (Lipitor, Crestor, Vytorin, Zetia/Ezetimibe, fluticasone propionate, Celebrex),

✪ Some antacids (Prevacid)

✪ Some general anesthetics (Halothane)

✪ Many antidepressants (Lexapro, Prozac) Toby Rogers wrote a poetic article HERE about how the toxicity of Prozac is related to fluoride.

✪ At least one non-steroidal anti-inflammatory or NSAID (S-Flurbiprofen)

✪ The benzodiazepine flurazepam (Dalmane)

✪ Antipsychotics (Risperidone, fluphenazine)

✪ Nasal spray allergy treatment (Flonase)

✪ HIV protease inhibitors, including tipranavir

✪ Cipro and Levaquin antibiotics. These carry a black box warning about some of the toxicities and must be avoided unless there are no alternatives.

Fluoride allows these drugs to cross the vascular barrier and into the brain. Although this is an advantage in treating brain infections, it can cause harmful mental effects.

Even traditional sources such as the *Merck Manual* acknowledge problems. It states:

Many newer fluoroquinolones have been withdrawn from the US market because of toxicity when given systemically; they include trovafloxacin (because of severe hepatic toxicity), gatifloxacin (because of hypoglycemia and hyperglycemia; it is still available in the US as an ophthalmic preparation), grepafloxacin (because of cardiac toxicity), temafloxacin (because of acute renal failure, hepatotoxicity, hemolytic anemia, coagulopathy, and hypoglycemia), and lomefloxacin, sparfloxacin, and enoxacin.

Fluorinated steroid creams are regarded as having little systemic (body-wide) toxicity. These include dexamethasone, triamcinolone acetonide, betamethasone, and beclomethasone.

"Citizen Zeus," who writes a Substack, says:

On May 1, 1999, Environment Protection Agency (EPA) scientists' National Treasury Employees Union published a devastating scientific article debunking fluoride use. They said it had no proven effectiveness and malignant, extreme harms. Their administrators disagreed and must have taken down the original link, for I had to go to the Wayback Machine HERE to find it. Excerpts follow:

Why EPA's headquarters union of scientists opposes fluoridation

by William Hirzy, PhD, [Union of Scientists] Senior Vice-President, Chapter 280

...Our opposition to drinking water fluoridation has grown, based on the scientific literature documenting the increasingly out-of-control exposures to fluoride, the lack of benefit to dental health from ingestion of fluoride and the hazards to human health. These include acute toxic hazards such as to people with impaired kidney function, as well as chronic toxic hazards of gene mutations, cancer, reproductive effects, neurotoxicity, bone pathology, and dental fluorosis.

In support of this concern are results from two epidemiology studies from China that show decreases in I.Q. in children who get more fluoride than the control groups in each study. These decreases are about 5 to 10 I.Q. points in children aged 8 to 13.

Another troubling brain effect has recently surfaced: fluoride's interference with the pineal gland's function. This produces melatonin which, among other roles, mediates the body's internal clock, doing such things as governing the onset of puberty. Jennifer Luke has shown that fluoride accumulates in the pineal gland and inhibits its produc-

tion of melatonin. She showed in test animals that this inhibition causes an earlier onset of sexual maturity, an effect reported in humans as well in 1956...

EPA fired the Office of Drinking Water's chief toxicologist, Dr. William Marcus for refusing to remain silent on the cancer risk issue. [Marcus] brought a lawsuit against EPA, claiming that they fired him because of his fluoride work. Dr. Marcus won his lawsuit and is now back at EPA.

...[There is] data showing increases in osteosarcomas in young men in New Jersey, Washington, and Iowa based on their drinking fluoridated water. It was [Dr. Marcus's] analysis, repeated statements about all these and other incriminating cancer data, and his requests for an independent, unbiased evaluation of them that got Dr. Marcus fired.

Regarding the effectiveness of fluoride in reducing dental cavities, there has not been any double-blind study of fluoride's effectiveness as a caries preventative. There have been many, many small-scale, selective publications on this issue that proponents cite to justify fluoridation, but the largest and most comprehensive study, one done by dentists trained by the National Institute of Dental Research, on over 39,000 school children aged 5-17 years, shows no significant differences (in terms of decayed, missing and filled teeth) among caries [cavities] incidences in fluoridated, non-fluoridated and partially fluoridated communities. The latest publication on the fifty-year fluoridation experiment in two New York cities, Newburgh and Kingston, shows the same thing. The only significant difference in dental health between the two communities as a whole is that fluoridated Newburgh, N.Y., shows about twice the incidence of dental fluorosis (the first visible sign of fluoride chronic toxicity) than seen in non-fluoridated Kingston.

John Colquhoun's publication on this point of efficacy is especially important. He was Principal Dental Officer for Auckland, the largest city in New Zealand, and a staunch supporter of fluoridation—until he was given the task of looking at the world-wide data on fluoridation's effectiveness in preventing cavities. The paper is titled, 'Why I *changed My Mind About Water Fluoridation.' In it, Colquhoun provides details on how data were manipulated to support fluoridation in English-speaking countries, especially the U.S. and New Zealand. This paper explains why an ethical public health professional was compelled to make a 180-degree turn on fluoridation.*

...Mutation studies...show that fluoride can cause gene mutations in mammalian and lower-order tissues at fluoride concentrations esti-mated to be present in the mouth from fluoridated toothpaste. Further, there were tumors of the oral cavity seen in the NTP cancer study... further strengthening concern over the toxicity of topically applied fluoride.

So, in addition to our concern over the toxicity of fluoride, we note the uncontrolled – and apparently uncontrollable – exposures to fluo-ride that are occurring nationwide via drinking water, processed foods, fluoride pesticide residues, and dental care products... For govern-mental and other organizations to continue to push for more exposure in the face of current levels of over-exposure coupled with an increasing crescendo of adverse toxicity findings is irrational and irre-sponsible at best.

We have also taken a direct step to protect the [EPA] employees we represent from the risks of drinking fluo-ridated water...the union filed a grievance, asking that EPA provide un-fluoridated drinking water to its employees *(Yoho emphasis).*

The implications of these calculations for the general public are clear. Recent, peer-reviewed toxicity data, when applied to the EPA's standard method for controlling risks from toxic chemicals, require an immediate halt to the use of the nation's drinking water reservoirs as disposal sites for the toxic waste of the phosphate fertilizer industry.

Yoho commentary:

Rachel Levine, the first openly transgender four-star officer in the armed forces and now Assistant Secretary for Health, delayed the release of a detailed report proving that fluoride reduced children's IQs (reference, January 2023). An EPA lawsuit forced its release in March 2023.

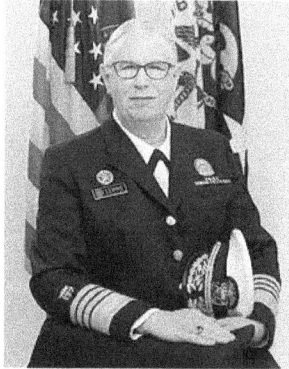

Levine

Chapter 11 explains why we are being subjected to fluoride. This is neither an accident nor incompetence.

References

Movies, academic studies, interviews, websites

The Fluoride Deception movie (28 minutes)

Fluoridealert.org (Fluoride Action Network)

The Case Against Fluoride (2010). Since it was published, more conclusive studies on neurotoxicity have come out. These include two NIH-funded long-term prospective cohort studies.

FluorideAction@FluorideAction

Here is some of the published science linking fluoridation to harm

Fluoride exposure and thyroid function among adults living in Canada: Effect modification by iodine status

A podcast where Christskis and Rivera, JAMA Pediatrics editors, discover that fluoride is harming our children's brains

FAN v EPA lawsuit

THIS is a fluoride toxicity Substack.

HERE is "Fluoride Free Australia."

"The Dangers of Fluoride" was the topic of Dr. Mercola's 2020 interview with Dr. Bill Osmunson. They discussed the studies showing that children who were exposed in utero to fluoride had lower IQs. Control groups from cities with no fluoridation had IQs that were about a standard deviation (15 points) higher. He described how the litigation to ban fluoride was being stalled.

Since the 1940s, when community water fluoridation was first initiated, fluoride and fluorine compounds were added to an array of consumer products... These include pharmaceutical drugs, carpets, cleaners, clothing, cookware, food packaging, paints, paper, and 16 other products. "Fluoride Consumer Products" is an academic article that you can download.

Truthaboutfluoride.com is a commercial site that sells products but is a source of independent testing and evaluation. I like it.

If you want to geek out about fluoride "controversies," THIS is a recording of the NTP BSC Fluoride Neurotoxicity Meeting from May 4, 2023. You can listen to how both the truth and the lies are presented.

Fluoride is *already* in our food and beverages.

Intended goal of fluoridation: Delivery of 1 milligram (mg) fluoride per day

Intended range of concentration in fluoridated water: 0.7 to 1.2 ppm
{Note: 1 mg (milligram)/Liter = 1ppm (parts per million)}

Fluoride Concentration, by specific independent analysis:
(Individual samples will vary)

Coca Cola Classic	0.98 ppm
Diet Coke	1.12 ppm
Sprite	0.72 ppm
Lucerne 2% Milk	0.72 ppm
Minute Maid orange juice	0.98 ppm
Gerber Graduate Berry Juice	3.0 ppm
Gerber White Grape Juice	6.8 ppm
Welch's White Grape Juice (concentrate)	1.8 ppm
Hawaiian Punch	0.85 ppm
Fruit Loops	2.1 ppm
General Mill's Wheaties	10.1 ppm
Kellogg's Shredded Wheat	9.4 ppm
Post's GrapeNuts cereal	6.4 ppm

Maximum allowable pesticide residue levels:
Cryolite (sodium aluminum fluoride)

Cabbage	45.00 ppm
Citrus fruits	95.00 ppm
Collards	35.00 ppm
Eggplant	30.00 ppm
Lettuce, head	180.00 ppm
Lettuce, leaf	40.00 ppm
Peaches	10.00 ppm
Potatoes, internal	2.00 ppm
Potatoes, wastes and skin	22.00 ppm
Raisins	55.00 ppm
Tomatoes	30.00 ppm
Tomato paste	45.00 ppm

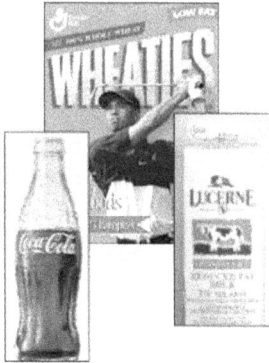

A bowl of Wheaties, a glass of milk, and a Coke or orange juice delivers twice the fluoride salesman's daily goal of fluoridation.

ITEM	FLUORIDE PPM	DOSE (MG)
12 oz. Coke	.98	.353
8 oz. 2% Milk	.72	.173
Wheaties	10	1.80
TOTAL DOSE		2.326

Exceeds 1.0 mg. Fluoridation Goal	1.0	**233%**

There is no deficiency of exposure to fluoride for any segment of our population.
Citizens for Safe Drinking Water • Jeff Green, Director • 1.800.728.3833

Chapter 9
Intermission: Three days living underground

Thirty years ago, I went miles underground into Lechuguilla Cave near Carlsbad Caverns. I stayed for three days, saw many places from THIS VIDEO, and swam across the underground lake.

The man who invited me on the expedition died last year of a vaccine-induced stroke. He was one of five of my friends who DFL to my advice and paid the ultimate price. It is beyond ironic that he took such care to climb and cave safely yet recklessly surrendered his body to public officials giving poisonous injections.

To my surviving friends: Please text me if you see this. If I never hear from you, I will know that you DFR my work.

If you have forgotten my acronyms, see post 211 in the RobertY oho.substack.com archives. The title is, "People do not freaking listen (DFL), even when their lives are on the line." Sign up for my blog while you are there.

I confess that sleeping and working inside caves for days on end freaked me out. I was always on the verge of telling my friends, "Let's get the f*** out of here."

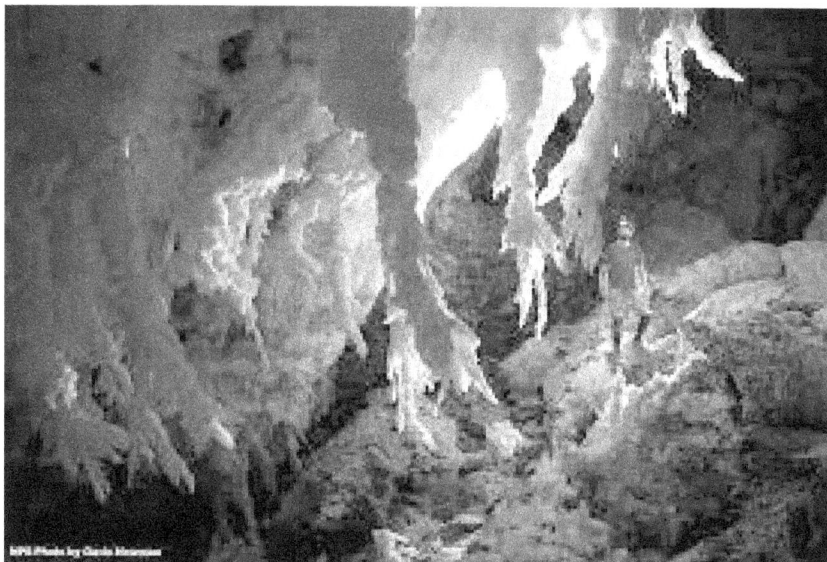

I saw this inside Lechuguilla. (Image from the video above.)

Chapter 10
Mark Kennard is the Canary in the Coal Mine

If you don't know, the thing to do is not to get scared, but to learn.

— Ayn Rand

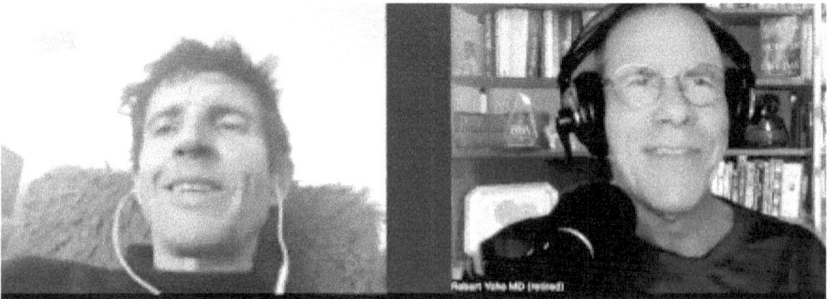

Mark Kennard/Robert Yoho

LINK. Rumble link HERE.

Mark is a brilliant person whose health problems have forced him to spend a decade researching. Because of his sensitivity to metals, his body violently rejects vaccines, dental work, and orthopedic implants.

Attempting to improve his health, Mr. Kennard studied metal toxicity and networked with international experts who tutored him. Although he is far more affected than most people, he has lessons for the rest of us.

Podiatrist Scott Schroeder became a metals authority when he saw patients like Mark. He says that dentists and orthopedists use implanted metals carelessly, but few doctors of medicine or dentistry are interested in hearing this.

Mr. Kennard says that any surgeon or dentist placing metal implants must test their patients before they operate. Very few of them do this now, and most do not even ask about the most common allergies. Many patients (17 percent for nickel) would admit, "Yes, I get a rash on my wrist where my watch touches," or "Cheap jewelry and I do not get along."

Even titanium, regarded by the mainstream as safe, has a reported allergy rate between .6 and 2.3 percent. However, the actual number is a multiple of this because orthopedic and dental titanium implants are alloyed with other metals. For example, the titanium used in dental implants usually contains aluminum and vanadium, which are linked to cytotoxic effects and allergies.

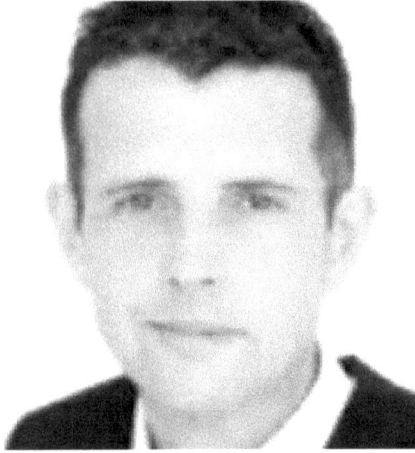

Mark in 2018.

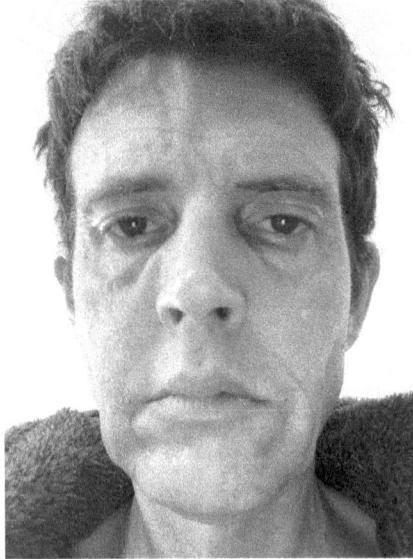

Four months later.

ABOVE ARE MARK'S PHOTOGRAPHS BEFORE AND AFTER THE implantation of orthopedic metals and aluminum-based bone cement. Mark: "That droopy face photo was taken four months after getting an implant with titanium screws and carbon fiber rods. I ended up being allergic to all of it."

Implants made of ceramics or having a nitride coating are available and less toxic. Custom implants can be made from other materials.

Mark also tells us how to detox safely and what the pitfalls are. Vitamin C is a wonder for health if you have no metals in your body, but he says it can speed up metal disintegration and toxicity if you are highly sensitive. Chelation to remove metals must be used cautiously and only by experienced practitioners. The top experts no longer recommend EDTA chelation for mercury because it potentially damages the kidneys.

Before my amalgam removal, Dr. Lagos drew blood to see if I would have problems with various dental composite filings that are available. I sent the report to Mark, and his comment made me wonder if I had moved too soon with my shoulder replacements:

Your report shows you have breached your mercury and aluminum antigen tolerance levels and that they will cause symptoms.

After you get your amalgams and other known sources of aluminum removed, your biggest problem will be your orthopedic implants. Their aluminum is your most significant threat to life and health. Finding more biocompatible implants is challenging.

Everyone implanted with metals will eventually become symptomatic and die. This happens sooner for people with specific gene mutations. Metals are the most challenging toxin for the body because they are solids that cannot be completely disposed of. Everyone chronically exposed to aluminum will eventually get Alzheimer's-type symptoms.

You are considering chelation or detoxification. Any process that speeds up the corrosion of your titanium alloy implants will release aluminum into your body. Slowing down its release buys you more time to be healthy and alive.

If your implants had no aluminum, you could go ahead and use products that speed up the detox process. But because there is aluminum in the shoulder implants, I recommend avoiding this unless you plan on replacing all your implants with new ones without aluminum. If the implants are left in, it's all about buying time.

Hopefully, your worst symptoms are caused by mercury. If so, all your health symptoms will vanish after your amalgams are removed. But this is unlikely. Symptoms from aluminum will not disappear unless you remove all of it.

I have a colleague who is an orthopedic implant surgeon. He and his partners have done thousands of knee and hip implants and have seen only a few issues like Mark's. Early in my friend's career, the implanted metals were more reactive, so the long-term results were less consistent. He says that today's titanium alloys with aluminum and vanadium have superior strength, biological compatibility, and wear characteristics. He reminded me that hip implants are recognized as the most successful surgery of the 20th Century. He writes:

Chromium cobalt (CrCo) implants have been used since the 1940s and were (and still are in some places) bonded to the bone using methyl methacrylate acrylic cement. CrCo alloys contain a small amount of nickel and are a source of what is thought to be true implant hypersensitivity reactions, yet they rarely require revisions. I've only seen two severe allergy cases in my career. Since many factors are in play for patients who require surgery due to implant failure, we have difficulty being sure about the cause(s).

Implants are structurally durable. They resist breakage and surface wear. Loosening at the bone interface after 10-20 years is the most common cause of failure.

Biological bonding, bone ingrowth into the implant texturing, is used for most modern implants. This eliminates the need for cement and reduces loosening over time as this "grout" fatigues and breaks down. Once ingrown, these self-repair through bone remodeling. Cement performs better, however, for the glenoid [the cup part of the shoulder joint]. CrCo is strong and inflexible (resisting breakage) but is affected by the implant material and bone elasticity mismatch. This may lead to atrophy and resorption of adjacent bone, which can produce bone loss, fatigue fractures, and loosening.

Commercially pure titanium, aluminum, and vanadium alloys with titanium or niobium have similar qualities as bone, so remodeling is more favorable and physiologically compatible. Like aircraft wings, they are fatigue-resistant under repetitive mechanical stress. Unfortunately, pure titanium is not as strong, and even its alloys, though stronger, have poor bearing surface wear characteristics. To improve this, they must be altered with nitriding, ceramic coating, and other methods. These add expense, alter biocompatibility, and likely have other long-term issues.

Metal-on-metal (MOM) hip implants were used between about 2004 and 2012. These created metal ion shedding and debris. For some people, it was directly toxic. The design of the implants seemed to be as important as the materials used.

About 70% of MOM hips are still OK and seem to last indefinitely, whereas most conventional metal or ceramic on polyethylene bearings will fail within 20 years in active patients. The most modern polyethylene is inert and durable, but we only have about 20 years of data. It is the most common material currently used in hip, knee, shoulder, and other implants.

Particulates related to wear, loosening, or implant breakage are generated by polyethylene, cement, or even implant texture fragmentation. This shedding causes tissue reactions in every patient to some degree. Metal ions (chromium, cobalt, and aluminum) may be directly toxic. Foreign body reactions (anything of a certain particle size and amount, including cement and ceramic debris) or allergies (typically nickel) are also possible.

Distinguishing between occult loosening and infection can be difficult in mild cases.

Infection and bearing surface failure are the most common issues that require hip and knee revisions. After ten years, two to four percent of patients need revision after primary cases, and twice that many for revision cases.

As a practicing surgeon, the usual problem is deciding when to re-operate on previously implanted people who develop pain. If it happens quickly—within three to four years after hip replacement—we have a diagnostic dilemma without definitive tests to guide us. Even if we know an allergy is involved, whether to operate may be unclear. Hip revisions are big surgeries with significant risks, and many people tolerate low-grade pain and do well long-term with the help of ibuprofen* or Tylenol.**

We do bloodwork, serum ions, joint aspiration, and imaging, but these are often inconclusive. X-rays might eventually show changes, but this could take six to eighteen months. We all hate to subject patients to a procedure that may not improve his status. But if we wait, we could be liable for a missed diagnosis.

Vast numbers of implants are placed, so allergy and sensitivity problems are significant and certainly under-appreciated. I doubt if one orthopedist in a thousand knows about the electrical currents between metals inside the body. I understand their viewpoint—they manage a spectrum of clinical problems and have trouble sorting out the importance of each one.

Allergy testing before surgery would improve informed consent and is a low price for better outcomes.

I have been asked whether I would have had my titanium alloy and chrome shoulder implants done if I had known then what I know now. I am not sure. My pain was tolerable before the procedure, but I have no pain now. But several years later, I am weaker, and despite weight training, I cannot fully regain my strength. Maybe I am just getting old.

Mark has given me doubts about how metals will impact my long-term health. If a patient asked me whether he should have implant surgery, I would tell him he has to make his own decision after he does his research. I would also quote J. Carl Cook: "Minor surgery is surgery someone else is having."

Postscript: Mark has a lot in common with the prescription drug-damaged people on Tim Alexander's "Legal Death" Facebook site.

Tim was propelled into action by his family connection to the San Bernadino killer, who turned violent because of psychiatric drugs. Mark and the people Tim studied had crippling reactions to toxic substances prescribed by doctors. These are well-known but little discussed. I told Tim's story HERE.

*Ibuprofen and other NSAIDs hinder bone growth.

**Tylenol depletes glutathione. According to Paul Thomas, MD, it should never be used and disposed of in a biohazard container.

References

HERE is an academic paper by Prof Vera Stejskal about the MELISA metals allergy assay (Also see MELISA.org).

Orthopedicanalysis.com is a related test performed in the USA. They do the metal-Lymphocyte Transformation Test (metal-LTT) that measures the amount of a cellular immune response called "delayed-type hypersensitivity."

Widespread testing would reveal people who are likely to have the most problems.

For metals geeks: Download "A comprehensive summary of disease variants implicated in metal allergy."

You can also follow the same metal allergy Facebook groups as Mark:

- Implant Allergy Support Group
- Hip Replacement and Recovery
- Breast Implants Can Kill
- Mercury Poisoning & Heavy Metal Detox
- Total Hip Replacement News

Chapter 11
Rebecca Dutton: the Protector-Goddess of People Damaged by Metals

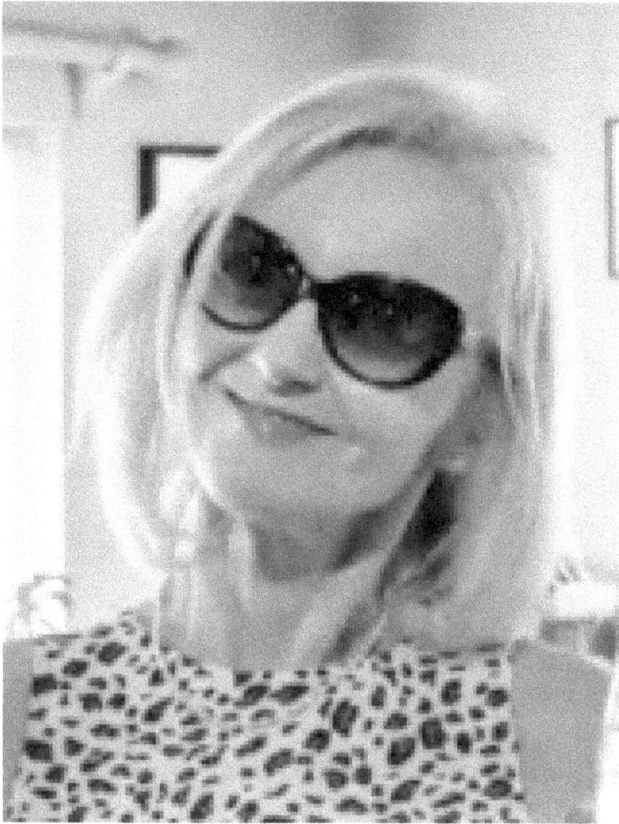

Here is Ms. Dutton at her recent 35th birthday party. Like her cousin Benjamin Button, she is aging backward.

LINK

Ms. Dutton has spent 16 years working with people damaged by metals and leads support and counseling groups. The average patient in Becky's practice has 12 to 16 amalgams. She makes no money from her efforts and lives in Stratford-upon-Avon, UK.

She has witnessed MS and other diseases heal after removing metals, particularly mercury amalgams. I am hoping this helps with my newly diagnosed Parkinson's disease.

Mark Kennard wrote: "I'm happy you've contacted Becky. She's one of the most knowledgeable and experienced people on the planet about mercury and diagnosing and managing type 4 metal allergy. She's the volunteer scoliosis researcher for MELISA.org, an allergy testing company."

Becky tells her story:

I worked in dentistry during the 1970's and was occupationally exposed to mercury. My daughter was exposed to mercury in utero and developed a neural tube defect and scoliosis. When I was diagnosed with chronic mercury toxicity in 2004, I received IV therapy to remove mercury from my intracellular pathways and DNA.

In 2007, I set up my first website, mercurymadness.org, and a support group. In 2008, I set up understandingscoliosis.org with Madeleine Holt, the former Culture Correspondent of BBC Newsnight. Then, Professor Vera Stejskal invited me to join the Melisa Diagnostics team (www.melisa.org) in 2011.

In 2014, I was appointed the lead UK activist for the Global Minamata Treaty to ban mercury pollution. One of the successful outcomes of our efforts was the new EU regulation to ban dental amalgam use in children under 15 and pregnant and nursing women. This came into force in July 2018 in the 28 EU countries, including the UK.

I developed robust evidence of the link between mercury exposure and scoliosis. This included studies of scoliotic fish living in mercury-contaminated water. In 2018, I was asked to speak at a conference in London, "Systemic Effects of Metal Exposure in Clinical Practice:

Protecting Patients and Optimising Outcomes." My presentation was 'Scoliosis, Spinal Surgery, and Metal Allergy.' It was about my research study of 66 people and the link between mercury and their scoliosis.

Dutton was treated to remove mercury from her body.

Mercury is primarily deposited in the brain and kidneys and is excreted mostly via the urine and feces. Although the biological half-life of mercury is estimated to be approximately 30 to 60 days in the body, the half-life of mercury in the brain may be as long as 20 years! Here is Becky:

I started IV therapy with hefty doses of vitamin C in February 2005. My doctor also prescribed vitamin and mineral supplements, a special diet, etc. I was advised to have all my amalgam fillings removed to complete the detoxification.

Immediately before and during my amalgam removals, I had IV vitamin C infusions followed by glutathione. With my vast occupational exposure, I may have been lucky not to have adverse effects from this. Another factor against me was having no gallbladder. This is one of the major detoxification organs.

A UK mercury-free dentist removed my twelve amalgam fillings and the piece of amalgam in my jawbone over ten days. During this period, I continued chelation with intravenous vitamin C and glutathione. When I passed urine, I could smell metal!

In 2010, I had monthly treatments with intravenous phosphatidyl-choline, folinic acid, and glutathione. These removed mercury, aluminium, and organophosphates from my DNA and intracellular pathways.

Toxins cause Parkinson's and related syndromes

After eight to ten years of a hand tremor, a neurologist diagnosed me with Parkinson's disease (PD). It is only a mild problem, but these things progress.

PD is the second most common neurological problem after Alzheimer's. It is a syndrome or constellation of signs and symptoms rather than a disease with characteristic lab tests. The cause(s) are not acknowledged by mainstream medicine.

Ken Stoller's book *Incurable Me* (2016) and my interviews with him convinced me that PD is closely related to autism, Alzheimer's, and Amyotrophic Lateral Sclerosis (ALS). I learned these are all due to or worsened by toxic exposures. A senior biological dentist told me, "In my opinion, Parkinson's is caused by mercury or paraquat."

Likewise, overwhelming evidence links autism with vaccines containing mercury. So, my working self-diagnosis is mercury toxicity. I hope to improve in the months following the removal of my amalgams.

Ken's book describes his experience treating patients with Lyme and other diseases. He writes, "As has been frequently pointed out, 'it' is never just one thing, but mercury is a toxic linchpin when it comes to many neurodegenerative disorders and is certainly synergistic with other toxins, such as glyphosate."

Like 70 percent of US citizens, a test showed glyphosate in my urine. As RFK says, "glyphosate is everywhere." Until recently, it was used to suppress weeds during the growing season, but it is now sprayed on wheat and corn immediately before harvest to dry it rapidly. This practice has multiplied our exposure. See the end of this chapter for other reasons to eliminate American wheat from your diet.

Dr. Dietrich Klinghardt successfully treats autistic children by decreasing their toxic exposures. He refuses to see kids from families that do not first remediate their home's electric and magnetic fields (EMFs). To treat glyphosate exposure, he suggests taking a teaspoon of glycine powder twice daily for three to six months. This causes urinary excretion of the pesticide. HERE is one of his Mercola interviews about this.

I decreased my EMF exposure by ethernet-wiring my house and doing electrical work. I am sleeping better, and the Wizard of EMF is returning soon for another home visit to exorcise more ghosts. (See the post HERE if you have not heard about him.)

Aluminum has been convincingly proven to be the primary cause of Alzheimer's, and it is closely related to Parkinson's. I am pushing my body to excrete it by consuming silica water. This story is HERE.

Here is the Goddess's expert opinion about my case

You've had quite a considerable amount of metal exposure during your life. First, your mouth: Seventeen amalgam fillings are a lot of mercury. Children of the post-war years were exposed to excessive amounts of amalgam. It was the 'drill, fill, bill' era— dentists were paid for each tooth they filled.

Your dentist says you have a metal crown, and there's an amalgam under it? Are there any metal posts? This alone could be causing many of your problems. Metal crowns are usually bonded with nickel, so you have nickel against an amalgam (mercury, silver alloy, tin, possibly zinc/copper). A post would be stainless steel. The metal crown is next to amalgams, so there is a good chance of galvanic corrosion in your mouth.

Do you have any cavitations? [bony soft spots that are often infected and visible on x-rays]. If so, they must be drilled out. [Not that I know about.]

You need to strengthen/treat your gut before your dental treatment. An anti-fungal diet and prebiotics/probiotics would help.

If you have clips in your knees, they are likely to be stainless steel, which has several metals. [I investigated and learned they were titanium alloy.]

Please find out the type of mesh used to repair your hernia. [There are hundreds of kinds, and they are plastic or polypropylene, not metal. There is only one exception, which is titanium.]

Do you have more details about the shoulder implants? [Titanium alloy and chromium, another alloy.]

You've smoked in the past; cigarettes contain several metals, including cadmium and mercury. [I caught this disease from my climbing buddy, Herb. Thanks, dude!]

You've had the flu vaccine. Depending on the manufacturer, Thimerosal, a mercury preservative, is still used in some vials. When you have the flu vaccine next time, please ask your doctor to check for Thimerosal. If it does, please refuse the vaccine because it has ethyl mercury!! [I would rather jump off a bridge than have any vaccine ever again.]

Thimerosal was in the contact lens solution you used many years ago.

Mercury is an endocrine disruptor that could have affected your levels of testosterone. [I had low testosterone levels and started replacement in my 40s.]

Removing amalgams and other dental metals should reduce your metal exposure and any possible galvanic reaction between the different metals in your body.

The best next step is phosphatidylcholine (PC) to eliminate the toxins remaining in your tissues. This, folinic acid, and glutathione, used intravenously in that order, remove mercury and other metals safely and effectively. Oral PC is available from BodyBio.com and works more gradually. I have observed many people while taking this, and their symptoms and laboratory tests improved dramatically. Some have had success with a teaspoon daily, but up to a tablespoon twice a day can be taken if tolerated.

Samuel Johnson noted, "When a man knows he is to be hanged in a fortnight, it concentrates his mind wonderfully." I am studying with a new sense of urgency and taking what actions I can. As my friend BCC taught me, "When your life is on the line, the best strategy is to throw all your hand grenades out at once." I remember his lessons and am doing my best to follow them.

References and Notes

From Dutton:

✪ Email Becky for a consultation: beckydutton@understand-ingscoliosis.org.

✪ Mercurymadness.org and www.UnderstandingScoliosis.org.

✪ The Symptoms of Mercury Toxicity summary sheet can be downloaded here.

✪ MELISA allergies testing website: Melisa.org.

✪ A summary video of a 2018 conference about metal toxicity is HERE. You can view the whole conference for about $30. I did and recommend it.

✪ HERE is Ms. Dutton's presentation about how mercury causes scoliosis. She cites both animal and human studies. In the UK, scoliosis rates rose as amalgams became more commonly used. Surgery has never been proven to reduce pain, improve lung function, eliminate spinal curvature, or correct rib and torso deformities. Implanted metals are toxic. Few patients are tested for metal sensitivity before these procedures.

From other sources:

✪ My German detox clinic doctor wrote me that the cumulative phosphatidylcholine needed to begin removing toxins effectively is about 0.5- 0.7 grams per kilogram of body weight. Oral and intravenous both count toward this total. He and his wife are healthy, but they still take a 2600 mg (2.6 grams) teaspoon of the BodyBio product daily. I am 80 kg, so 56 teaspoons (18 tablespoons) are needed to get .7 grams per kg. I have taken more than this over the past month.

✪ "Meta-analysis of Metal Allergies" by KA Roach & JR Roberts (2022) is everything we know about metal sensitivities. Download

✪ Mercury Toxicity: How It Hides In Your Food & Poisons Your

Health by Dr. Mark Hyman is a video summary of the clinical problems with mercury. He had mercury toxicity that he says was treated successfully with dimercaptosuccinic acid (DMSA) chelation.

Boyd Haley, a University of Kentucky chemistry professor, is an expert on this subject. He says that DMSA and 2,3-Dimercapto-1-propanesulfonic acid (DMPS), another substance used to treat heavy metals, should not be used to remove mercury. DMSA removes mercury from the blood and concentrates it in the kidneys, which can cause renal failure. Also, most mercury is not in blood but inside cells. According to Dr. Haley, neither DMPS nor DMSA can enter the cell, so these only remove mercury from the blood.

Appendix: Recommended protocols during dental amalgam removal

From a DDS senior IAOMT member:

IV C is good for everything. It cancels local anesthetic, so do it after the removal or during. I recommend the "SMART protocol IAOMT method" to minimize risks.

Glutathione is depleted in almost everyone who has amalgams because mercury releases iron inside the mitochondria, leading to oxidative stress, cancers, and aging. Glutathione is made inside the mitochondria to protect you from the oxidation that creates energy. That is the electron transport system. Mercury releases iron inside mitochondria and produces free radicals that cause oxidative stress.

This rapidly uses up your glutathione, and aging, fatigue, and ill health results. There is 1000 times more glutathione inside the mitochondria than in blood. Once in the bloodstream, it is rapidly excreted.

Oral glutathione is digested before absorption. IV can circulate and potentially clean toxins from blood but will never get through the blood-brain barrier due to its charge. It cannot get into mitochondria, so until mercury exposure stops, healing cannot begin.

So yes to IV C and ok IV glutathione when you are getting amalgam removal, but first and foremost, minimize exposures.

Airway protection with separate air sources for patients and doctors is vital.

From another DDS IAOMT member:

All the havoc mercury causes in the organs and other parts of the body is impressive and frightening at the same time.

Is there any part where it doesn't cause harm? I doubt it.

We always give IV vitamin C. The amount depends on the patient's weight and underlying health issues. Typically, we give 0.75 grams per kg bodyweight during the procedure. After the vitamin C is finished, we give 600mg glutathione IV push.

Vitamin C has benefits for the detox process. With seventeen amalgam fillings, I would use all the gear available to support their removal and detox. Vitamin C and glutathione are essential.

We also suggest a pre-removal supplementation protocol that uses liposomal vitamin C, glutathione,* selenium, and multiple daily mouthwashes with activated charcoal to gather the released mercury.

Ken Stoller, MD

Protocol:

❂ *Eat a diet high in proteins and vegetables for two weeks before your procedure.*

❂ *Ensure that you have one to two bowel movements per day. Magnesium citrate suspension can be added to water, tea, or juice, one or two tablespoons daily, to induce the two bowel movements. Be sure to drink lots of water. Use half of your weight in pounds in ounces per day, divided over your waking hours, such as four ounces or a cup of drinking water each hour you are awake. You can also add ground or powdered flaxseed to your drinks or foods like sauces, cereals, or salads (one or two heaping tablespoons daily) to induce two bowel movements daily.*

❂ *For three days before amalgams are removed, take • Chlorella, 1 gram three times a day • Vitamin C, 1 gram three times a day • Cilantro, 1 gram three times a day • Glutathione 3,000 mg* (bonus to take garlic with this as well)*

✪ *Before going to the dentist, take 3,000 mg (3 g) of chlorella and 3,000 mg (3 g) of vitamin C.*

✪ *The dentist should provide oxygen by mask or nasal cannula so that you do not breathe in the toxic gas that comes out of your mouth as he drills out the amalgam filling. The dentist should also use a coarse bit that breaks up the amalgam into chunks rather than a delicate bit that pulverizes the amalgam, which can spread and penetrate more easily. He should use a high-volume suction apparatus and a rubber dam to reduce your exposure to toxic particulates.*

✪ *Chlorella dissolved in the rinse water and sprayed in the mouth helps reduce exposure during the procedure. Eye protection is also provided to the patient to avoid exposure through the conjunctiva. The dentist and her assistant should use a gas mask and eye protection to protect themselves from the toxic fumes, and the procedure should be performed in a room that does not circulate air into the rest of the office. The room should be separately vented and have appropriate filtration to trap mercury released from drilling. An anionic air-purifying device in the room may also be helpful. The dentist should use a lot of water, chlorella rinse, and spray to bind the mercury and reduce exposure.*

✪ *Based on the dentist's preference and experience, only one quadrant or less should be removed at a time unless the fillings are small.*

✪ *Once your amalgams are out, we can consider chelation and supplements that boost your detox.*

✪ *Use oral NAC and glutathione* until your amalgams are out.*

*To repeat, respected sources say oral glutathione is poorly absorbed.

Part Two

Judas Dentists Live Inside the Rockefeller Medicine Matrix

Chapter 12
"Almost Everything Scares Me These Days."

We are fast approaching the stage of the ultimate inversion: the stage where the government is free to do anything it pleases while the citizens may act only by permission; which is the stage of the darkest periods of human history, the stage of rule by brute force.

— Ayn Rand (1905-1982)

LINK

Apanoply of health risks are being forced on us. These are used to make money, injure us, and make us die sooner. Most can be avoided. This chapter synthesizes brutal information, so here is some lighter fare.

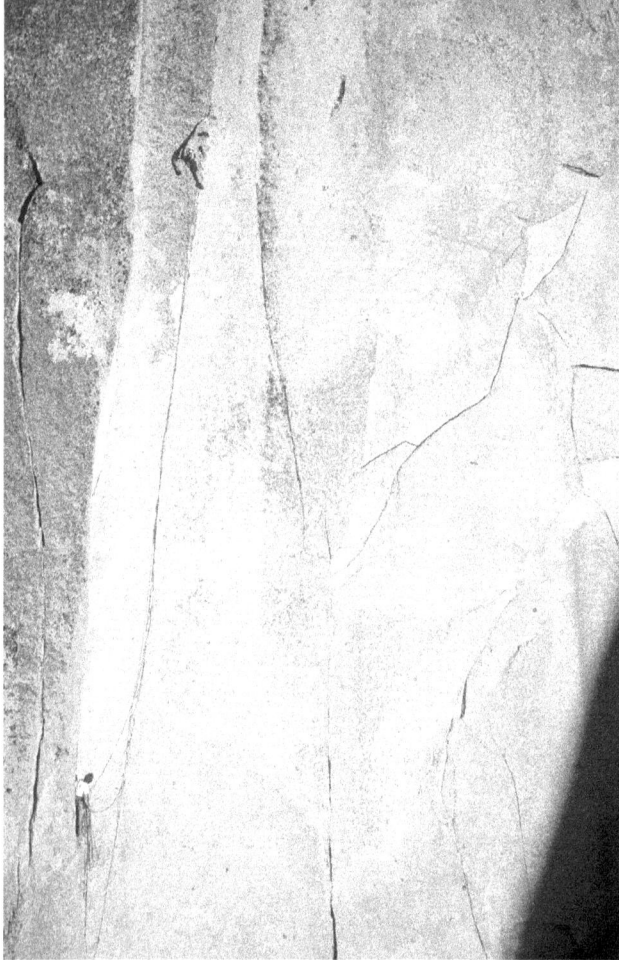

We were once young and heedless. (Needles photo credit: Kris Solem)

This chapter's title is what Dick Cilley, my "dirtbag" climber friend, continuously chanted while scaling hazardous rock. We would gleefully repeat his words as we ascended, laughing at the situations we put ourselves in.

A quote often attributed to Julius Caesar explains more, "As a rule, what is out of sight disturbs men's minds more seriously than what they see." The dangers I describe here are mostly invisible, so our anxiety about them may be higher than they merit.

The worst risks are self-imposed

Climbing is hazardous, but smoking is responsible for one in five US deaths. I spent a magic decade of my life doing these simultaneously.

A "conventional" source lists the most common causes of US deaths in 2021:

1. Heart disease 695 k
2. Cancer 605 k
3. Covid 416 k
4. Accidents 225 k
5. Stroke 162 k
6. Alzheimer's 119 k
7. Diabetes 103 k

You can avoid most of these

Strokes and heart attacks increase if you eat "unsaturated" vegetable fats like Crisco or margarine. These oxidize, which causes diabetes, atherosclerosis, and other damage. Since the early 20th century, industrial food producers and a paid-off American Dietary Association have claimed these cheap synthetics are healthy. "Saturated" animal fats, on the other hand, oxidize much less, so they promote good health (Hormone Secrets).

Eating seed oils instead of animal fats is being recognized as another cardiovascular health catastrophe. Big agriculture, fast food restaurants, fake fat makers, and corrupt regulatory groups are co-conspirators in bringing these to us.

Avoiding exercise creates similar risks as smoking.

Accidents: Auto accidents kill 43,000 Americans annually. Not wearing a seatbelt doubles this risk.

Suicide: 50,000 in the US yearly. The psych drugs cause much of it and should be outlawed because of this and other reasons.

"Covid deaths" is code for *people slaughtered by the Covid bioweapon, those killed by withholding standard therapies, those killed by the vax, and those murdered by doctors with treatments such as Remdesivir, fentanyl, and ventilators.* It was all facilitated by CDC and FDA lies and implemented by the Department of Defense. If you understand this story, you can save yourself and your family.

How to escape modern health calamities

Studying increases your chances of survival. Never be accused of DFR or DFL (don't freaking read or don't freaking listen).

Some of the following disasters are forced on us; others are caused by suppressing or concealing effective treatments. For example, iodine restriction is obviously purposeful. For the rest, ask yourself, "Could this have been solely caused by chance, greed, or incompetence?" The answer is mostly "No."

The following hazards are in rough order of death and disability rates.

Medical abuses

These are the use of therapies that do not work, cause active harm, or for which simpler, safer, or more effective alternatives are available. At least half of modern medicine is abusive, and some of the most significant risks are on this list. *Butchered by "Healthcare"* tells more. (For clarity, I put some into separate categories below.)

How did it all happen? The beginning was when Frederick

Gates, henchman for John D. Rockefeller, guided the writing of the *Flexner Report* (1910). This directed medicine's path into the 21st century and was the start of Rockefeller's destruction of its integrity.

Medical "errors." These are deviations from mainstream "standards of care" that cause harm. A credible study estimates that this causes 250,000 US deaths a year.

Prescription drugs kill 250,000 yearly in the US and Europe, according to Peter C. Gøtzsche. This is the third most common cause of death after heart disease and cancer.

The psych drugs. These cause violence, suicide, and early death. Twenty-five percent of Americans and 80 percent of Danes have been convinced to use them. They destroy our health, empathy, and humanity and are phenomenally addictive. RFK, Jr. forced Fauci to admit in writing that they had never been studied against placebos. This means the "science" behind them is a tissue of fraud.

Cancer cures. Dozens of safe, cheap, and effective treatments have been suppressed. For example, double-blind, placebo-controlled studies have proven that solid tumors respond to mistletoe. Fenbendazole, a drug related to ivermectin and sometimes used in combination with it, is cheap, nontoxic, and avidly suppresses lymphomas.

Chemotherapy. A few lymphomas, testicular cancers, and other tumors can be successfully treated. However, the oncologists who reviewed decades of published studies report that their poisons improve patient survival by an average of less than two months. It is an admission of utter failure for treatments that cost $100,000 or more a year. Radiation therapy is less successful than chemo, for it does not even produce this statistically invisible outcome for any disease except prostate cancer.

The oncos are paid well to fail; they get 25 percent kickbacks on the chemo charges for the drugs they administer. If doctors paid each other off like this, it is "capping," a felony. (*Butchered by "Healthcare."*)

Root canals (medical subcategory)

These spread infection through the body and must be removed if you value your health. Its inventors repudiated the procedure, but it is still universally performed by general dentists and endodontists. About half of the people in the developed world have these inside their mouths. Root canals cause a double-digit percentage of all human diseases in developed countries, possibly as much as 40%.

Vaccines (medical subcategory)

Without exception, each is a net harm that creates illness, shortens lifespan, and decreases fertility. These cause more damage than other drugs because "medical standards" allege they are safe and effective and should be forced on all of us many times, starting at birth. They contain mercury, aluminum, and other toxins that destroy health.

Notes:

✪ Except for the (totally ineffective) influenza vaccine, none has contained mercury for two decades. But since mercury takes years to leave the body—if it ever does—vaccinations are still the second largest human exposure after dental fillings.

✪ Before the Covid jab, most immunizations were injected by bribed pediatricians. Over the last few decades, childhood vaccines caused the autism rate to rise from 1/10,000 to 1/30.

✪ No vaccine has ever been studied using a saline placebo comparison. This would have been performed and published if the vaxes worked.

✪ The Covid jab has no medical utility. Worldwide death rates soared within months after its rollout, and live births plummeted. This proves it is a bioweapon developed to weaken and kill us.

Dental amalgam poisoning (medical subcategory)

These are a more significant source of mercury than vaccines. They initially contain 54 percent, and they dissolve and release it into the victim's body over many years. Amalgams are marketed as "silver fillings" by ignorant, unscrupulous dentists. They are a pre-Civil War technology that puts a volatile, malignant toxin into the most reactive part of the human body.

Comment

Dentists have no pretense of following even the ruined science of mainstream medicine. They regard themselves as mouth carpenters rather than physicians responsible for a sensitive biological system.

When they "drilled, filled, and billed" my 17 amalgams, I was too young to say no. The mercury likely caused Parkinson's, gave me scoliosis, and affected my personality. Dentists have damaged most of you as well.

Watch Dustin Hoffman in Marathon Man HERE (three minutes) to witness dental sadism. Robert Gammal says this type of cruelty is real. You will think this is gratuitous only if you are new to the study of dentistry.

Opioid abuse and overdose deaths (medical subcategory)

This is being thrust on us from the outside. The "physician standards" were altered, and predatory, opportunistic doctor prescribing contributed. Overdoses now slaughter over 100,000 US citizens a year.

Bioidentical hormone suppression (medical subcategory)

Medical standards for hormone prescribing are a pack of FDA lies and defamations. Doctors seldom prescribe these because their bribed academics discourage it.

Few seniors take them, and most of those who do receive inadequate doses. Bioidentical hormones, the only ones worth considering, prevent premature aging and extend healthy lifespans. Their use preserves muscles, intellect, and emotional stability. But they are under assault.

Testosterone was placed on the scheduled drug list despite its negligible toxicity and profound benefits. Contrary to censored sources like Wikipedia, it benefits the heart. It can also cure advanced breast cancer. See *Hormone Secrets* for more.

Aluminium

This is the second most toxic metal to which humans are commonly exposed. Fortunately, you can mostly avoid it and force its elimination from your body if you read and listen to my Substack posts HERE and HERE.

Electromagnetic fields (EMFs)

These come from cell phones, WiFi, and unshielded wiring sources. The dangers are better recognized in Russia and Europe than in the US. Our knowledge is limited because the telecom juggernaut suppresses research and information flow.

Some people cannot tolerate EMF. To mitigate it, WiFi can be replaced with ethernet wiring, which is safer and faster. But solutions like these are ignored in the quest for sales and convenience. The result? We now bathe in electrical fields. But with care and study, we can decrease our exposure.

EMF may deserve a higher place on this list. See my posts HERE, HERE, and HERE.

Fluoride poisoning

This neurotoxin is deliberately placed into US, Australian, Canadian, and other water supplies. Studies prove that babies born to mothers who consume it have lower IQs. Industrial fluoride producers give the American Dental Association millions yearly to promote this poison as a tooth strengthener. Agents of the Biden cartel continue to block ongoing lawsuits against its use.

The vegan cult promotion

In November 1944, Donald Watson coined the word "vegan" after watching a pig get slaughtered. He defined it as never consuming animal products. Never in history, before or since, has any large group eaten only plants and retained their health. The oft-cited contrary examples, such as India, are *vegetarians* who also use eggs, dairy, and sometimes even fish. US vegans are the biggest group, but to survive, most of them cycle in and out of strict compliance. Overwhelming evidence has developed that this cult practice damages its adherents over the long run.

But Gates, the World Health Organization, and the captured media support it—and these people are eugenicists. Those who are fooled by them blindly damage their health. See Hormone Secrets and THIS post.

Lyme disease (medical subcategory)

Like syphilis, this is a spirochete, and ticks spread the infection. It was developed as a bioweapon by our government, then released upon our children and us. The evidence for this includes the deathbed confession of Willy Burgdorfer, Lyme's most prominent researcher.

Lyme has chronic, insidious symptoms. It is hard for "mainstream" doctors to diagnose and treat because knowledge of the natural history and therapies is suppressed. But there are many promising "alternative" treatments, including hyperbaric oxygen, chlorine dioxide, and Alinia, an anti-parasite drug that can be used off-label.

Infected ticks are now ubiquitous in wooded areas of the US and parts of Europe. Ken Stoller estimates that a mid-double-digit percentage of American citizens have been exposed. Most of the symptomatic ones have no idea what is wrong with them. If not recognized and adequately addressed, Lyme can cause profound disability. See Chapter 15.

Sun exposure suppression and sunscreen promotion (medical subcategory)

This is a bizarre dermatology psych-op that lined their pockets and damaged anyone who believed them. It started when a Madison Avenue marketing company told the Derm leaders to change their image from foolish pimple poppers to fierce cancer fighters.

Skin docs were soon charging millions a year for office cancer checks and pricey "skin surgeries" that could sometimes be performed with nail clippers. They developed the "standard" that every bit of skin removed must be inspected under the microscope and a substantial charge generated. They began using the same type of billing codes that surgical pathologists employ when examining systemic cancers. (Question: Which breed of doctor makes the most money? See * below.)

The truth about the sun was sacrificed to marketing lies. Contrary to what the dermoids** claim, sun exposure is profoundly healthy—if you have the minimal level of judgment required to avoid roasting yourself. Consider:

✪ Women who are outside regularly have a far lower risk of breast cancer than those who avoid the sun.

✪ Safe, regular sun exposure can eliminate or reduce depression.

✪ We are told that melanoma incidence has multiplied even in this era of sunscreen and sun avoidance. But this is dishonest reporting; the proper measure, melanoma deaths, has remained the same.

✪ The dermatologists use this lie to make us afraid of even walking outside. They recommend instead that we scurry into their offices clutching our hats and have "suspicious lesions" clipped off at great expense.

✪ Cancers, heart disease, autoimmune diseases, the flu, Parkinson's, multiple sclerosis, and infertility are reduced by sun exposure.

✪ Sun exposure increases the likelihood of a healthy pregnancy and baby.

✪ Women who get sun have only one-eleventh the risk of a hip fracture as those who do not.

✪ Sun avoidance and using sunscreen might be as hazardous as smoking.

See The Sunlight Institute website for references and more.

*Answer: A few dermatologic pathologists have gross billings of $40 million annually.

** A dermoid is a cyst filled with stinky dead skin; it is also my pet name for dermatologists. I know about dermoids because I spent a year in one of their training programs. To my credit, they fired me, and you can read about it in *Butchered by "Healthcare."*

Ivermectin suppression (medical subcategory)

If used correctly, ivermectin would have saved millions of lives from Covid, even without other treatments such as vitamin D and chlorine dioxide. But during the initial "pandemic," a massive publicity campaign branded it as "horse medication." This was used to discredit this safe, effective, Nobel Prize-winning medication.

Hydroxychloroquine (Plaquenil) suppression (medical subcategory)

This nontoxic drug has been used since 1955 to treat inflammatory autoimmune diseases. Although patients typically take it safely for decades with little monitoring except for eye exams every six months, sources such as the CIA-run Wikipedia claim its side effects are severe. A study in the Lancet "proved" it did not help Covid, but the paper was withdrawn after it was outed as a fraud two weeks after publication.

Suppression of Vitamin D and other supplements (medical subcategory)

D is the most crucial nutrient for good health, but the doses available have been deceptively altered to cut consumption. The units used to measure it were changed from (the tiny-sounding) micrograms to "International Units (IUs)," which are measured by the (perceptually huge) ten-thousands. The commonly available doses are 1,000 to 5,000 IUs, but we now have 50,000 IU capsules, which can be taken once or twice weekly. Some people must take them daily to keep their levels adequate for good health. These are the same size as the ones containing 1000 to 5000 IU of D.

The National Institute of Health claims that 20 ng/ml vitamin D levels are "adequate for most people." However, people who have levels over 60 rarely get Covid and other viral illnesses. Levels of 100 may be healthier.

Zinc, quercetin, and vitamin K2 can successfully treat and prevent deaths from viral illnesses such as Covid. This has also been suppressed.

Iodine has been recognized to promote health for more than a century. A program to discredit it and substitute toxic alternatives such as bromide has been ongoing for about 20 years (Chapter 13).

The US RDA (Recommended Daily Allowance) and other

sources claim we need little or no vitamin C, magnesium, zinc, selenium, thiamine, and boron. The wonderfully therapeutic effects of large Vitamins D, C, and magnesium doses are suppressed or ignored. These three and others, such as thiamine and sometimes hydrocortisone, should be given intravenously to nearly every sick hospitalized patient, but they are not.

Aspartame (NutraSweet, Equal) promotion

This artificial sweetener is still available everywhere. A review says, "Dozens of studies have linked aspartame—the world's most widely used artificial sweetener—to serious health problems, including cancer, cardiovascular disease, Alzheimer's disease, seizures, stroke, and dementia, as well as negative effects such as intestinal dysbiosis, mood disorders, headaches, and migraines... [plus] weight gain, increased appetite, and obesity-related diseases."

Chlorine dioxide suppression

This may be the most important story on this list. Read about it HERE in the archives of RobertYoho.substack.com or in the last chapter of this book.

Heedless use of industrial toxins

Since the 1950s, industrial toxins have been inserted into our food, medicines, and myriad commercial products. Left unsaid were the long-term consequences. Some of these hazards were unknown at the start, but they were deliberately hidden later. These include DDT, glyphosate, paraquat, Agent Orange, trichloroethylene, and heavy metals such as mercury. Due to these and others, neurological diseases such as ALS, autism, Alzheimer's, and Parkinson's redoubled over the past few decades.

Glyphosate herbicide is used universally in the US even though it causes cancer and creates dependence on psychopathic agricultural corporations. It is mostly banned in Europe. Taking chlorine dioxide dissolves it (see Chapter 16). Dr. Klinghardt says you can make your body excrete it by taking powdered glycine daily. He describes how to reduce other hazards as well.

Cut your risks

Your health is not due to random chance. It is your body's precious natural immunity minus all its toxic exposures. Mark Kennard explains how it works in a five-minute video HERE. He says stresses are additive and describes how you will get sick if you cross your resistance threshold. Healing yourself might be as easy as adding one supplement or decreasing a single toxin, but functioning at your best may require many changes. Words to this effect should be in the preface of every functional medicine book.

Almost everything still scares me these days, but I know how to avoid dangers. If you listen and read, you will, too.

No one is coming to save you

Although some of this has to be greed or incompetence, we have overwhelming proof that malign hands directed the rest. Joe Plummer's *Tragedy and Hope 101* is a history of how the globalists created disasters to weaken and destroy us. They stay hidden, for they fear exposure.

When I tabulated these calamities

I was repeatedly stunned by physicians' central role and systematic collusion with the criminals. I was also shocked anew by the conspiracy's scope and organization and by how many weapons had been deployed against us.

As I uncovered story after story of physicians' ethical perversions,

I recalled Cicero's maxim: "Nothing is so strongly fortified that it cannot be taken with money." Businesspeople understand this, but physicians, trained more like academics, always pretend their behavior is kosher.

Litigation is beating back some of it, but this is sluggish and unreliable, so you must take matters into your own hands. The first step is to realize that nearly every public story we hear is a lie. Learn as much as possible, change your thinking, and correct what you can.

Reservoirs of strength remain to us, and we have hope. Our bodies are so resilient that our death rate never increased until we allowed poisonous needles to be thrust into us. John Dryden's words about his battle apply to ours: *I am sore wounded but not slain. I will lay me down and bleed a while, and then rise up to fight again.*

History teaches us that leaders appear when times are the most desperate. Dire need and the press of events forge these people. We are witnessing it now.

The rest of us must use the time we have to spread the truth and expose the criminals. As long as we are living and breathing, we can do more. We just have to be strong enough.

Aurelius again

Work steadily at that which is before you, following right reason seriously, vigorously, calmly, allowing nothing to distract you, but keeping your divine part pure, as if thou shouldst be bound to give it up immediately. If thou holdest to this, expecting nothing, fearing nothing, but with the heroic truth in every word and sound you utter, then you will live happy. And there is no man who is able to prevent this.

Chapter 13
Iodine is Vital and It Has Been Taken From Us

W hen heroes are needed, courageous journalists and doctors answer the call.

Hero #1: Lynne Farrow

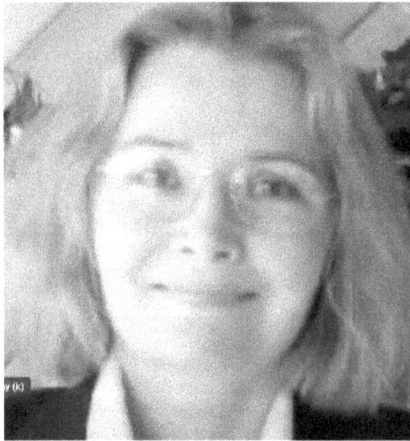

Ms. Farrow tells how the vital iodine supplement used in bread was systematically replaced with bromide, a toxic waste. It is a dark story, but the good news is that if you educate yourself, you can easily take enough iodine to improve your health. HERE is one of Lynne's presentations.

LINK

Lynne's book, *The Iodine Crisis: What You Don't Know About Iodine Can Wreck Your Life*, was published in 2014 and recently revised.

Farrow was never healthy, but when she was diagnosed with breast cancer, she started researching wholesome living. She writes:

Fear can make you jump onto the first available treatment conveyor belt and plod through the steps assigned to you, no questions asked. Worse, fear can make you believe in the six most dangerous words in the English language, "They must know what they're doing." Those six words sustained me for about a month. Got cancer? Step one. Find a well-known doctor at a major Metropolitan hospital. Done. Dr. B. was smart, kind, personable, detail-oriented, and open to my endless questions. You would think this partnership between patient and doctor would work out great, right? Well, no, and yes. My relationship with the famous surgeon worked out fine right up to the point when she lied to me ...

Lynne soon became more knowledgeable than her physicians. For example:

At a local cancer conference, I asked a question of the doctor who served as Director of Breast Cancer Services at one of the country's foremost cancer hospitals. "Does radiation therapy increase overall survival in breast cancer patients?" I asked this question because I had researched the medical literature and already knew the answer—No. I was testing him to see if his information was reliable. His response: "Radiation must increase survival because we do it at our hospital."

In her quest to understand and cure her breast cancer, Ms. Farrow eventually stumbled onto iodine, a critical trace element. She began studying its background and uses. It had a venerable history spanning thousands of years. Until the antibiotic era, it was regarded as a top disease prevention and treatment method. It was painted on the skin as a disinfectant, used to treat breast diseases, and placed on wounds to counter infections. Taken internally, it was known to produce healthy teeth, nails, and hair. It is essential for proper energy, sexuality, thyroid health, and more.

Since the body cannot produce iodine, it must be consumed. Lynne learned that iodine availability had been systematically curtailed since the 1970s. Although you can still buy iodized salt, up to 90 percent of the supplement evaporates rapidly once a package is opened. Also, this type of salt is more difficult to absorb than when the nutrient is supplemented in foods. Iodized salt is just enough to prevent goiter but insufficient for optimal health. It also contains aluminum, which promotes Alzheimer's and Parkinson's Disease.

Until recently, bread was fortified with iodine. But as Lynne writes, "A 1970 conference report from the Food and Nutrition Board, National Academy of Sciences [NAS], titled 'Iodine Nutriture in the United States,' strongly hinted that iodine in bread may not be safe and that iodized salt is superior... The function of the report appears to be to raise insidious questions disguised as public concern—Is iodate in bread dangerous?"

In *Hormone Secrets*, I wrote about when, a few years ago, the Academy was contracted to discredit bio-identical hormones made by compounding pharmacies. It was a pay-for-play hatchet job. The purpose seemed to have been to eliminate one of big Pharma's tiny competitors. I concluded that the prestigious NAS was as full of whores as the rest of medical academics. Before I read Lynne's book, I had no idea they were this corrupt in 1970.

Lynne continues, "By 1980, wild claims were published. The USDA [United States Department of Agriculture] reported in "The Fortification of Foods: A Review" that iodine as a disinfectant 'has long been known to be lethal...' and that Americans get more than enough iodine from non-bread sources, so [iodine] 'should be replaced whenever possible by compounds containing less or no iodine.'"

In 1973, potassium bromate, a toxic anti-iodine, was substituted for the iodine formerly used in bread. This purged the critical nutrient from our bodies. The UK banned this practice in 1990, and Canada did the same in 1994, but in the US, petitions to the FDA to eliminate bromate have been unsuccessful.

Within a few years, bromines added to fire retardants increased our exposure to the toxin. Lynne wrote, "Fire retardant dust is the most grievous source of bromine; countless other sources flow into our bodies from brominated vegetable oil in certain sodas, sports drinks, and foods. We are surrounded by bromine and bromides, an insidious element known to sedate, suppress the thyroid, disrupt reproduction, and even cause mental illness. Bromine fire retardants are even found in breast milk. Bromide is banned in many countries but not in the US."

Breast cancer rates have risen since the 1970s. During the same period, as iodine consumption decreased, exposure to bromine increased. IQs are dropping, and thyroid and other diseases continue to worsen. Obesity is partly due to the iodine metabolic pathways being poisoned with bromine.

Fluoridated drinking water, ubiquitous in the US but banned in most of the world, also decreases iodine absorption.

Large Chinese population studies have shown that iodine deficiency causes dwarfism, poor thyroid function, and mental retardation. In some cases, this has been corrected with supplementation and dosing iodine using crop irrigation.

Low iodine consumption causes more problems for women than men because pregnancy and nursing require extra iodine. The following stories from Ms. Farrow's book describe how deficient women respond to supplementation. They suddenly feel great—sometimes on the first day. These are from LynneFarrow.net:

Patient story, Alice: breast calcifications, coldness, hair loss, Raynaud's Disease, all improving or resolved.

I started using iodine about 18 months ago when I decided not to get a stereotactic biopsy for suspicious calcifications. I took an iodine loading test. I was only slightly deficient, about 15 percent, but the doctor advised me to take 100 mg daily of Iodoral along with ATP cofactors in case of an early stage of cancer. About six months ago, I had an ultrasound of the area, and after careful examination, there were no visible calcifications. I did not get a mammogram as I did not want to have one anymore, but I knew that the calcifications picked up on my last mammogram had also been seen on the ultrasound. Also, thermographs showed improvement and less inflammation in the area.

Iodine has done wonders for me. Fibrocystic disease is clearing up. I also may have had a sluggish thyroid that was not picked up on blood tests, as now my feet are no longer cold, my Raynaud's Disease has gone away, and my alopecia (hair loss) is almost resolved. I am taking 50 mg of Iodoral a day, and my fibrocystic disease may take another few years to resolve completely. I took other measures I researched, but I think the Iodoral was the main player in my success. I hope my story helps others.

Patient story, Marla: Lumpy, sore, fibrocystic breasts resolve. Energy improves.

I want to tell you about my experiences with Iodoral. It has been the most beneficial product I have ever used. I have fibrocystic breasts, which my gyno simply described as "lumpy, sore breasts." He said it really doesn't hurt you; it just hurts. Well, I think that is bull. I started doing some research on my own and ended up going to a chiro for a back problem. She had me lie on my stomach to adjust me, and, wow, did my breasts hurt! Well, that was the best day of my "health" life! My husband was the first to link a difference to the Iodoral. In about three weeks, I just felt good. Really good. I had energy; I felt like going places and doing things. It was not a jittery caffeine energy; it was just what a normal 30-year-old should feel like. And my libido was back. That is what my husband noticed! Before the Iodoral, I didn't want to be with my husband. But suddenly, I wanted to! And finally, on to my breast. My breast pain would start exactly ten days before my period. And be very severe. In the second month, no pain. None at all. And it doesn't come back as long as I am on my Iodoral. If I am not on it, it comes back immediately. My mother had breast cancer at 38. I am now 35, I have taken control of my health, and I will not be a silent victim!

Hero #2: David Brownstein, MD.

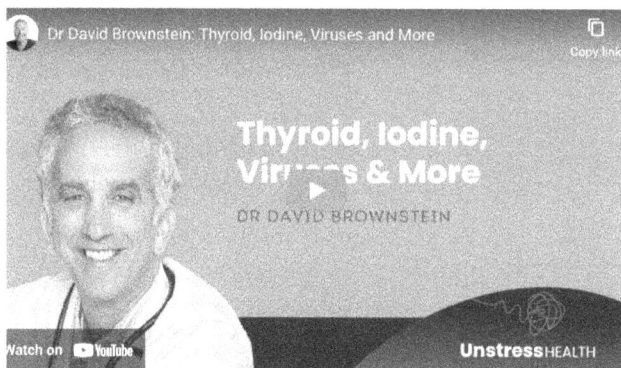

Dr. David Brownstein: Thyroid, Iodine, Viruses and More

This 2022 podcast is an interview with David Brownstein, MD., author of the 2014 book *Iodine: Why You Need It, Why You Can't Live Without It* (the paperback costs $43, but the ebook is available HERE for $15). Listen to it at faster speeds. HERE is another of the doctor's podcasts.

Dr. Brownstein describes how he quit conventional medicine and became an expert in nutrition, bio-identical hormones, and other holistic therapies. He has lectured internationally and written sixteen books.

Brownstein says people who live near the ocean or who eat a lot of fish get plenty of iodine. However, his Midwest area is known as the "goiter belt" because the soil is iodine deficient. So he helped develop a test for it and found that seventy percent of his patients had low iodine levels. When given iodine, a third can stop their thyroid medication, a third can reduce it, and only a third must continue at the same dose.

He says that if he had to leave functional medicine and use only one of his therapies, he would keep iodine because it helps the most people. In the video above, he also addresses fluoride, thyroid, and hormones. He describes why, contrary to accepted medical "wisdom," there is a general salt or sodium chloride deficiency.

Four "halides" are important for humans—(sodium) chloride, fluoride, bromide, and iodine. Our levels of chloride* and iodine are grossly deficient, and we are being poisoned with fluoride in the water and bromide from many consumer products. Fortunately, if we take adequate iodine, it displaces bromide from our tissues and forces its urinary excretion. Unfortunately, this may not be the case for fluoride. *See the Appendix below.

Brownstein says we must do our homework for health issues. His motto is, "The best-educated patients get the best results."

What we can learn from censored sources

Although mistakes are often made in science and medicine, the following lends credibility to the idea that globalists are guiding the mainstream iodine narrative. For example, Wikipedia's article "Iodine (medical use)" contains none of this information. WebMD's write-up had none, either. It has been censored since it was sold to a huge investment firm in 2017. A third, Healthline, has the biased title, "Ten Uses for Iodine: Do Benefits Outweigh the Risks?" It says:

Given the wide availability of iodine in Western diets, thyroid health isn't typically impacted by low iodine levels in the United States... Despite the role iodine can play in disinfecting drinking water, there are also some concerns that it can increase the total iodine intake in humans and lead to adverse health effects (Yoho note: this is unreferenced). *Total iodine intake shouldn't exceed 2 mg per day* (This cites NIH sources, which are certainly captured).

The iodine truther community says twelve-and-a-half to fifty mg daily is the optimal dose of iodine for normal people. As Lynne learned with her breast cancer, glandular tumors such as breast, prostate, and thyroid can sometimes be suppressed using several hundred milligrams daily. But for most people, Dr. Brownstein recommends starting with 25 mg every morning. See the references and the dosing recommendations below to learn more.

Should you simply buy some iodine and start taking it? On a hazard-to-benefit ratio, it seems like an excellent idea. If you take too little, it works poorly, and if you take too much, it gets excreted in the urine if your kidney function is normal. The only problem that occasionally occurs is getting "hyper" or "revved up." Savvy patients rely on their personal responses to adjust their doses.

Feeling better can be nearly instantaneous or take weeks. If you have thyroid issues, seek supervision from an experienced practitioner who knows about iodine. Brownstein says that he can successfully manage Graves and Hashimoto's thyroid diseases using larger doses of iodine.

He rarely resorts to radioactive iodine, which is the "standard of care" for these conditions. This is used to partially or wholly destroy these diseases' hyperactive thyroid, but it unfortunately spreads throughout the body and causes long-term damage.

I had a formal consultation about my health with Dr. Ken Stoller. Among other things, he recommended a drop of "nascent" iodine every morning. That set me on the path to reading all I could and writing this. I was soon taking six drops daily, and later increased my dose to 50 milligrams a day of other types.

It is disgraceful that this knowledge is not a part of standard medical training and practice.

Dosing

Several types of iodine are available. The bioavailability of each medication that follows is different, so the ideal milligram doses are not precisely equivalent. Also, people have different needs for iodine because some are deficient, and some are not.

✪ Lugol's solution was developed in 1829. Two drops of Lugol's 5% Solution contain the equivalent of one tablet of Iodoral 12.5 mg.

✪ Lugol's as a 12.5 mg pill: Iodoral brand from Optimex contains 5 mg iodine and 7.5 mg potassium iodide. The doses recommended by some holistic doctors are 25 to 50 mg each morning.

✪ Nascent (the Magnascent brand and others) was developed in the 1920s. It is more expensive and has a reputation for greater purity and reliability. There are 400 micrograms or .4 mg per drop. This is a tiny dose, but if you are deficient, a few drops will dramatically affect you. I started slow and increased the amount I took.

✪ SSKI (saturated solution potassium iodide) was developed in the 1800s and has 0.05 grams (50 mg) per .05 milliliter drop. A milliliter is a full gram, and a third of a milliliter is about 300 mg.

Lynne emailed me this concluding comment: "I don't think you can overdo iodine unless you're feeling bad and then 'that's the bromide talking.'" She learned this through 15 years of study and interacting with online groups. Getting your dose right is an adjustment process that you should not rush. Read a lot and get knowledgeable help if you can find it. My Substack readers had more subjective improvement from iodine than anything else I wrote about.

References

Look at Lynne's book (cited above) first because of its readability and fascinating story. It sold over a million copies and has been translated into eight languages. Also see:

✪ www.BreastCancerChoices.org and LynneFarrow.net. Her Breast Cancer Think Tank is HERE. Iodine is one of their recommended strategies. She is also the editor of Iodineresearch.com.

✪ At the Yahoo iodine group, you can learn from beginners, practitioners, and long-time iodine takers HERE (accessed through the Wayback Machine).

✪ The Curezone Iodine Forum HERE (accessed through the Wayback) is managed by its founders, Laura and Steve. They have had over 10 million hits.

✪ *Iodine: Why You Need It, Why You Can't Live Without It* (2014) by David Brownstein, MD. He has YouTube videos, a website, and many books on Amazon.

✪ THIS reference is about the epidemic of iodine deficiency in US women of reproductive age.

Experts to consult

There are many others.

✪ David Brownstein, MD (rumored not to be taking new patients, but you can try)

✪ Ken Stoller, MD

✪ Margaret Aranda, MD

✪ Lynn Farrow recommends Dr. Buist, an expert holistic doctor in Wyoming, Michigan. Her websites are NaturalThyroidChoices.com and SteppingStonesLiving.com.

Appendix: more Brownstein

One of Dr. Brownstein's most interesting insights was that the 1997 INTERSALT World Health Organization (WHO) study recommending low salt consumption for high blood pressure was wrong. It was a demographic study comparing population groups. These are some of the weakest "science" in medicine, and the authors purposefully threw away most of their data to obtain the wrong conclusion. These days, everything WHO is suspect, but this was before we knew about it.

Brownstein advises his patients, including hypertensives, to take several teaspoons of yellowish, unrefined sea salt daily. He recommends the Redmond or Celtic brands, which contain critical trace minerals. Unfortunately, the reverse-osmosis process commonly used to eliminate fluoride removes these from household drinking water, so we need to supplement.

Dr. Brownstein says salt improves patient health and does not raise blood pressure. HERE is the link to his book, and HERE is an interview.

During the first Covid wave, Brownstein prescribed the same treatment protocol he used during the prior flu seasons:

✪ Vitamin A, 100,000 U a day

✪ Vitamin D, 50,000 IU a day

✪ Vitamin C, 1000 mg an hour orally at first

✪ Iodine 25 to 50 mg a day

✪ Inhalant nebulizers with .03 percent hydrogen peroxide (diluted from 3 percent) and one drop of Lugol's iodine in the solution. It is used every two hours at first.

✪ Intravenous vitamin C is given to sicker patients.

Dr. Brownstein spoke about his therapies in this podcast, Redefining Medicine, with special guest Dr. David Brownstein.

His practice treated thousands of Covid patients, and only one died. Brownstein's partner sent the man to a hospital, and the doctors there murdered him with Remdesivir. If you think this statement is over-the-top, listen to any of Scott Schara's interviews in my archives. THIS is one.

My friend George had this to say about Brownstein's protocol, "I'm just getting over the worst summer flu/Covid that I've ever had. I have been gargling and nebulizing povidine iodine for several days, which immediately made a difference. I am mega-dosing on vitamin C powder as well."

For more, HERE is a podcast Brownstein did with Mercola. It was primarily about the viral treatment protocol above.

Parting Shots

Iodine and boron are vital:

#1. Jorge Flechas, MD, MPH, wrote, "We know from world studies that if you give iodine during pregnancy, the babies that come out are usually 20-30 points higher in IQ than their parents." HERE is his speech explaining how iodine is critically important for women and the elderly to avoid cancer and other health issues.

#2. For accidental or wartime radiation exposure, adults of eighteen and older should take 130 mg of iodine a few hours before or as soon as possible after the event, then daily. This is two ccs of KI (potassium iodide) solution.

#3. The boron suppression story HERE is similar to iodine's.

Chapter 14
Intermission: After you climb El Cap, everything else seems easy

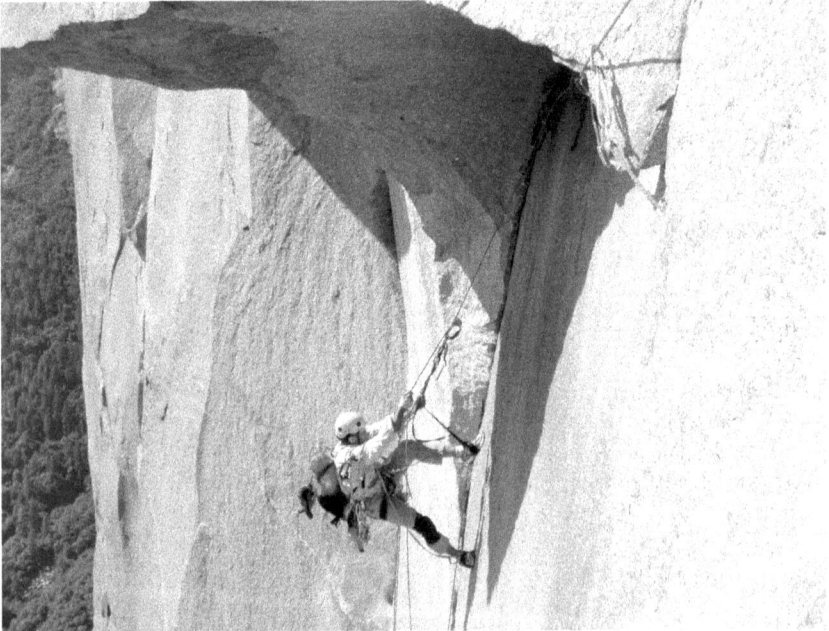

It was one of the best days of my life. I was 53 and ascending Yosemite's El Capitan in 10 hours with climbing hero Hans Florine. This is halfway up, under the Great Roof.

Chapter 15
Like Covid, Lyme Disease is a Bioweapon

Lyme has infected a double-digit percent of the world's people, and effective treatments are being hidden. It was deployed against us from a US military research lab on Plum Island, Connecticut, in 1975.

LINK

I was introduced to Lyme when I was 26 and in a Dartmouth dermatology residency. We were all fascinated by this new disease and its "target" skin rash. The dermatologists dubbed it "erythema chronicum migrans" to baffle other doctors and hog the stylish new condition for themselves. I saw a few cases that looked like this:

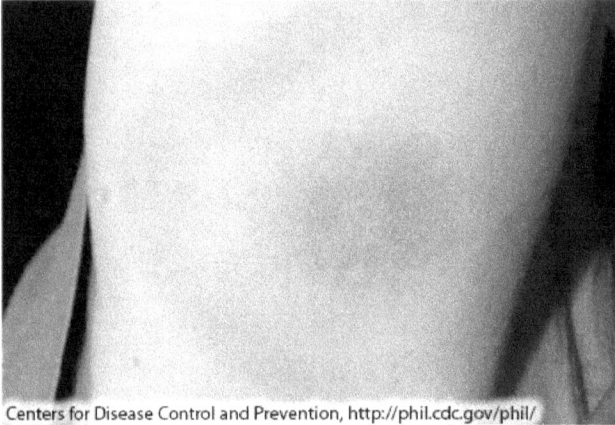

Centers for Disease Control and Prevention, http://phil.cdc.gov/phil/

My dermatology training consisted of endless, picayune academics. I only wanted to climb the New Hampshire mountains to rock climb and hike the Appalachian Trail. When the dermoids discovered my attitude, they kicked me out of the program. I thought this was a catastrophe.

Here is the CDC's description of Lyme:

[It] *is the most common vector-borne disease in the United States. Lyme disease is caused by the bacterium Borrelia burgdorferi and, rarely, Borrelia mayonii. It is transmitted to humans through the bite of infected black-legged ticks. Typical symptoms include fever, headache, fatigue, and a characteristic skin rash... Infection can spread to joints, the heart, and the nervous system if left untreated. Lyme disease is diagnosed based on symptoms, physical findings (e.g., rash), and the possibility of exposure to infected ticks. Laboratory testing is helpful if used correctly and performed with validated methods. Most cases of Lyme disease can be treated successfully with a few weeks of antibiotics. Preventing Lyme disease includes using insect repellent, removing ticks promptly, applying pesticides, and reducing tick habi-*

tat. *The ticks that transmit Lyme disease can occasionally transmit other tickborne diseases.*

The rest of this chapter is from a post written by "Unbekoming," an anonymous commentator. Oscar Wilde wrote, "Imitation is the sincerest form of flattery." I take my admiration to extremes; For essential material like this, I occasionally rewrite someone else's work like a respectful editor. Whoever this guy is, I cannot keep up with him. His original essay is HERE.

"Ticks have a special place in my heart," by Unbekoming

We live in St Ives, one of the tick capitals of Sydney, Australia. When we bought the house, I remember the real estate agent telling us all the amazing features of the suburb (they were all true), but he left out the ticks…

So, for the last 20 years, we have accumulated tick stories. Our kids and cats were regularly bitten and treated. Our most serious story happened when my wife was bitten by a small army of ticks and was unwell for several months. She "luckily" came down with a kidney stone, so the hospital flushed her with IV antibiotics and inadvertently killed whatever infection she had picked up from the ticks. Thank God for the kidney stone, I guess.

The daughter of a friend contracted Lyme disease but couldn't get a doctor in Australia to diagnose it. She was forced to travel to the US to work with a doctor who helped her treat it over a long period.

It never crossed my mind, not even for a second, that anyone would have spent decades trying to figure out how to weaponize ticks with all manner of bacteria and viruses. But that's precisely what they did.

I remember telling my wife that the tic design was simply perfect. They would crawl up your leg without you knowing and burrow into your skin to secrete their toxins and drink your blood. By the time you felt them, it was too late.

In the 1940s, the US military decided that tics were perfectly designed for what they needed to do.

One of the reasons I think the tick and Lyme story is so important is because it, via Newby's book, Bitten, *supplies a window straight into who "they" are—the book names names.*

How Lyme came to Unbekoming's attention

Toby Rogers put Lyme on my radar as a bioweapon when I read THIS post in September 2022:

Having Lyme, ME/CFS, or an autoimmune disorder is like wearing an electric dog shock collar that you cannot take off. Every time you try to engage with the world, the thing shocks you, and you're worse off than if you had not tried at all. Over the years, it has created learned helplessness. What's troubling to me, especially given the history of Lyme (it's likely an American-made bioweapon), is that governments highly desire the ability to create learned helplessness in a population. The peasants cannot overthrow the feudal system if they wear biological shock collars that constrain their ability to dream, think, and act. We have got to find ways to cure these conditions. Healing is a revolutionary act.

In July 2023, I read Denis Rancourt's essay:

I do not mean that the Department of Defense (DoD) does not fund gain-of-function and bioweapon research (abroad, in particular); I do not mean that there are not many US patents for genetically modified microbial organisms having potential military applications. I do not mean that there have not previously been impactful escapes or releases of bioweapon vectors and pathogens. For example, the Lyme disease controversy in the USA may be an example of a bioweapon leak. See Kris Newby's 2019 book, *Bitten: the Secret History of Lyme Disease and Biological Weapons* [894 Amazon reviews].

I find ticks and Lyme easy to understand because I study other US government "theatrical productions." These include AIDS, smallpox, fluoride, Covid, Covid vaccines, DDT, polio, glyphosate, and childhood vaccines. This background, plus Rancourt's article quoted above, jolted me into writing the following book summary.

Unbekoming outlines *Bitten*

The US military:

✪ Weaponized ticks.

✪ Used those weaponized ticks on foreign soil against both military personnel and civilians.

✪ Engaged in uncontrolled releases on US soil.

✪ A "mysterious" new disease emerged.

✪ Willy Burgdorfer, a scientist, purportedly discovered its connection to ticks. He was hailed as a hero.

✪ Turns out Willy was one of the lead scientists who, years earlier, had weaponized the ticks (you can't make this stuff up).

✪ The US medical establishment denied the existence of the new disease and attacked the doctors who diagnosed or tried to treat it.

✪ The medical industry now profits from Lyme.

Unbekoming quotes from *Bitten:*

✪ Reported cases of Lyme disease have quadrupled in the United States since the 1990s. In 2017, 42,743 cases of Lyme disease were reported to the Centers for Disease Control and Prevention (CDC). The scientists at the CDC who study the spread of diseases now say that the actual number of cases may be ten times higher than reported, or 427,430 cases. On average, this means there are about 1,000 new Lyme cases in the United States per day.

✪ While all the pieces of this public-facing story are true, they are not the whole truth. Shortly before his death, Willy was videotaped saying that he believed that the outbreak of tick-borne diseases that started near Lyme, Connecticut, had been a bioweapons release.9 It was a stunning admission, but it could explain why the condition we call Lyme disease is so hard to diagnose and treat—and why the epidemic is spreading so far and so fast.

If anyone else had said this, I might have walked away, but Willy was the person with the most to lose. When this information came to light, his legacy would be destroyed. Because of this horrible secret, the foundational science behind Lyme disease was compromised, and patients were being harmed.

✪ Willy learned that a lab full of researchers who loved bugs was being funded primarily because of the government's need for disease vaccines. The US Public Health Service, which would later be renamed the National Institutes of Health, paid for the lab by developing, manufacturing, and distributing vaccines for spotted fever, encephalomyelitis, relapsing fever, yellow fever, and other diseases transmitted from animal or arthropod vectors to man.

✪ On a lab tour, Willy was told how the lab mass-produced ticks and Rickettsia rickettsii organisms to manufacture vaccines. In the 1920s, researchers there injected thousands of guinea pigs and rabbits with these live organisms, then placed ticks on the infected animals and allowed them to feed for a couple of days. They would then douse bacteria-laden ticks with formalin, grind them up, and use the filtered, diluted "tick juice" as a vaccine. The vaccine fluid included tiny fragments of proteins that, when injected under a person's skin, would stimulate a protective immune response.

✪ In her 2005 book, *Biological Weapons: From the Invention of State-Sponsored Programs to Contemporary Bioterrorism,* medical anthropologist Jeanne Guillemin, now a senior fellow in the Security Studies Program at the Massachusetts Institute of Technology, describes the political situation as Willy became one of the 13,538 civilian employees of the US chemical and biological weapons program: "The atomic bomb and the Cold War signaled a momentous change in the US biological weapons program. The vision of the scale of intentionally spreading disease expanded to strategic attacks on a par with the destruction of Hiroshima and Nagasaki and with the Soviet Union and its allies as potential targets."

✪ The army recruited young scientists such as Willy to staff this massive scientific effort, often funding them through the US Public Health Service (later the National Institutes of Health) and the National Academy of Sciences. The secrecy of these projects was modeled upon the strict guidelines developed for the Manhattan Project, whose scientists had had to sign confidentiality agreements and had not even been informed about the ultimate purpose behind their experiments: weapons development.

✪ There was a method behind this madness. In most cases, bacteria from one region wouldn't thrive inside ticks from another region because it takes many generations for a microbe and a tick species to develop a mutually beneficial relationship so one doesn't kill the other. When Willy found a compatible pair, Fort Detrick would add that agent/tick combination to its list of potential biological weapons. The weapons designers sought a tick that wouldn't arouse suspicion in an enemy country. They would infect it with an agent for which the target enemy population wouldn't have natural immunity.

✪ From Brigadier General Lansdale's Top-Secret Memorandum, January 19, 1962: "On a most discreet (strictly need-to-know) basis, defense is to submit a plan by February 2 on what it can do to put a majority of workers out of action, unable to work in the cane fields and sugar mills, for a significant period for the remainder of this harvest. It is suggested that such planning consider non-lethal [bioweapon], insect-borne.”

✪ From the Biological Subcommittee Munitions Advisory Group, October 27–28, 1966: “Dr. A. N. Gorelick reviewed the characteristics of viral and rickettsial agents currently in the program . . . the use of multiple agents to achieve prolonged incapacitation was also being investigated.”

✪ The perfect incapacitating agent made a large percentage of a population moderately ill for weeks to months. The illness it caused would have to be hard to diagnose and treat, and under the best circumstances, the target population shouldn’t even be aware they’d been dosed with a bioweapon. This would make it easier for invading, vaccinated soldiers to take over cities and industrial infrastructure without much of a fight or the destruction of property.

✪ According to the Infectious Diseases Society of America (IDSA) guidelines, chronic Lyme isn’t classified as an ongoing, persistent infection; it’s considered either an autoimmune syndrome (in which a body’s immune system attacks itself) or a psychological condition caused by “the aches and pains of daily living” or “prior traumatic psychological events.” Medical insurers may use guidelines like these to deny treatment, and many guideline authors are paid consulting fees to testify as expert witnesses defending denial of insurance coverage. In some states, guideline recommendations take on the force of law so that Lyme physicians who practice outside them are at risk of losing their medical licenses.

✪ Guideline authors regularly convened in government-funded, closed-door meetings with hidden agendas. These lined the pockets of academic researchers with significant commercial interests in Lyme disease tests and vaccines. Many government grants were awarded to the guideline authors and lab researchers.

✪ Over the years, the US military conducted “Large Area Coverage” vulnerability tests on an unsuspecting public. For example, in the 1950s, the US Navy sprayed a two-mile-long line of aerosolized “simulant” off the coast of San Francisco. In *Bitten*, Newby described the effectiveness of such an attack if the weather conditions were right.

✪ I pondered why Lyme disease researchers were much more paranoid than their rickettsial counterparts. Reflecting on my research for the Lyme documentary *Under Our Skin*, I concluded that much more money was at stake with Lyme disease. It was the first major new disease discovered after the Bayh-Dole Act, and the Diamond v. Chakrabarty Supreme Court decision made it possible for the NIH, the CDC, and universities to patent and profit from "ownership" of live organisms.

When the causative organism behind Lyme disease was announced, something akin to the Oklahoma Land Rush of 1889 began. Scientists within these institutions began furiously filing patents on the Lyme spirochete's DNA and surface proteins, hoping to profit from future vaccines and diagnostic tests that used these markers. For example, an NIH employee who patents a bacterial surface protein used in a commercial test kit or a vaccine could receive up to $150,000 in royalty payments a year, which might double his annual salary.

All of a sudden, the institutions that were supposed to be protectors of public health became business partners with Big Pharma. The university researchers who had previously shared information on dangerous emerging diseases were now delaying publishing their findings so they could become entrepreneurs and profit from patents through their university technology transfer groups. We lost our system of scientific checks and balances.

This undermined patients' trust in the institutions that are supposed to do no harm. With Lyme disease, there's no profit incentive to proactively treating someone with a few weeks of inexpensive, off-patent antibiotics. But the patentable vaccines and mandatory tests-before-treatment bring in steady revenues year after year.

✪ More than a decade after the tick bite that changed my life, I had a deeper understanding of the Lyme problem from a scientific, political, and policy point of view. I knew that infectious disease departments at most major medical centers were following the iron-fisted IDSA Lyme guidelines stating that chronic Lyme isn't an infectious disease and that it can't be successfully treated with long-term antibiotics. Even Stanford cooperated.

Back to Yoho: effective therapy is being concealed

If you think you have Lyme, you probably do. If you think Pfizer will save you with a vaccine, you also believe in the Easter Bunny. If you want to read fiction about Lyme's diagnosis and treatment, look at Wikipedia.

For better advice, contact Ken Stoller, MD. His interviews with me and his website are HERE and HERE. He says that a double-digit percentage of US citizens are infected. He makes it sound like this number is nearly on the order of root canal illness. How many are symptomatic is unknown. To treat the disease, Dr. Stoller uses hyperbaric oxygen and Alinia, a benign anti-parasite drug that you can buy over the counter from Indian pharmacies.

Chlorine dioxide solution (CDS) cures Lyme disease. It is cheap, safe, and easy to make. It is also heavily suppressed, which is clear evidence that it works. See the next chapter.

When Lyme spirochetes. die, toxins are released that can make you sick. This is the Herxheimer reaction; both Alinia and CDS can provoke it. Ken and other experienced doctors recognize this and can advise your therapy. Find a provider who is knowledgeable and motivated. Use low starting doses and be careful.

Reference

The Lyme documentary *Under Our Skin* (2008) "Exposes the hidden epidemic of Lyme disease and reveals how our corrupt healthcare system is failing to address one of the most serious illnesses of our time." It was censored off YouTube but is on Amazon Prime.

Chapter 16
Chlorine Dioxide is Kryptonite to Rockefeller "Healthcare"

Any sufficiently advanced technology is indistinguishable from magic.

— Arthur C. Clarke

LINK

To focus, I brush off 95 percent of the torrent passing before me. Chlorine dioxide (CD) was like that at first, but then a friend breathlessly recommended a video featuring an annoying German,* Andreas Kalcker. He said that CD cured everything from AIDS to cancer to every infectious disease. I loathe exaggerations; he spoke with ridiculous certainty, and—this is still a reflex for me!—he was only a Ph.D. It was three strikes against him.

*I can say this because I am German, too.

I can pry something understandable out of almost anything. But since I had cut most of my schoolboy chemistry classes and never studied electrical engineering, I had trouble with Kalcker. As I watched him at my usual double speed, I found nothing easily verifiable. So, I shelved the project, and months passed.

Then Christian Elliot sent me his Kalcker interview with a dozen links. As usual, I found myself racing to catch up. Christian could more easily approach the subject because he lacks my biases and thinks better than me.

I learned that NASA called CD a universal antidote and that it was a cheap, nontoxic, reliable disinfectant used widely since the 1970s. Hundreds of studies were published about its safety and efficacy. It has been used to treat species from humans to honeybees, which are profoundly sensitive. In humans, chlorine dioxide is a proven cure for many illnesses. For some animals, it improves longevity.

By 2006, information about CD began going viral. The buzz was that it was easy and cheap to make, cured many conditions, and no doctor was needed. In response, a massive government smear campaign was launched in 2010 that equated using chlorine dioxide with drinking bleach.

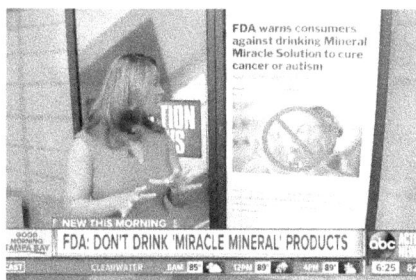

Idiot newscaster reading from a script about the supposed
horrors of chlorine dioxide.

My interest sharpened when I learned about this; it resembled
the ivermectin "horse medicine" lies. The psychopaths wanted us to
view CDS as a conspiracy.

As I explored further, I found "Chlorine Dioxide as an Alternative Treatment for COVID-19" and other similar sources. I also
heard reports of CD curing Lyme disease and autism. Sometimes, the
best path to the truth is reversing the lies from censored sources.
Wikipedia, which is CIA-sponsored, calls these claims lies.

Lyme and COVID were developed by the US government's
"gain of function" research labs to injure and kill us. Autism is caused
by childhood vaccines, which are proven killers and likely
bioweapons as well. The stories about CD being the same as bleach
and the "horse medicine" lies about ivermectin might have been
invented by the same advertising agency.

All this reflects years of planning. The criminals obviously realized that their plans were threatened if the word got out that chlorine
dioxide cured these diseases or that ivermectin healed Covid. To see
how their fear-mongering continues, search YouTube for "Church of
Bleach."

Chlorine dioxide is a nontoxic sanitizer with thousands of established uses.

It was first produced in 1811. Since then, myriad applications have been devised, including use in over 500 US water treatment facilities. It is not carcinogenic and is even used in fish tanks without harming the fish. In conventional dilutions, CD has no proven human or animal toxicity, even for people on the edge of death.

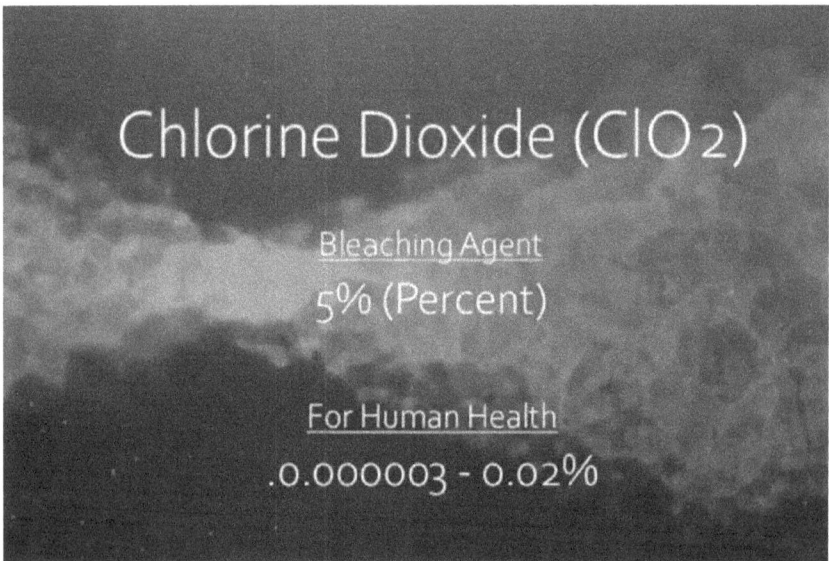

Chlorine Dioxide (ClO$_2$)

Bleaching Agent
5% (Percent)

For Human Health
.0.000003 - 0.02%

Chlorine dioxide is used for paper bleaching but in extreme concentrations and amounts that have nothing to do with human use.

CD may be the best-known disinfectant. It can eliminate bacteria, fungi, viruses, and tiny parasites. Extremely low doses are effective medical treatments, and no toxic metabolites exist.

Since it has so many important uses, it cannot be banned. And since it cannot be patented, making enough to last a lifetime costs under $100. It is easy to manufacture at home using sodium chlorite (not sodium chloride, salt) and an acid "activator." Hydrochloric acid 4 percent is best, but others are effective as well.

CD has been proven safe for consumption by humans at concentrations of 10-100 parts per million, even when used daily for months. It is pH neutral and does not typically cause irritation or other side effects.

Chlorine dioxide's safety trials are extensive and remain unchallenged. Viruses and bacteria are killed by tiny concentrations that host cells survive unharmed. We also have animal trials. In one, when mice were experimentally infected with influenza, all those exposed to low-dose chlorine dioxide lived, and 70 percent of the rest died.

Formal studies of CD treating and curing human disease are rare. The few accepted for publication claim near-universal clinical success within a day to a few days. However, the media has discredited and defamed this work and the authors. They even did this to Kalcker despite his impressive background.

How does chlorine dioxide work? Human cells can easily handle the oxidation produced by chlorine dioxide, but viruses and bacteria cannot, so they die. Kalcker says, "[CD] is oxidizing, which is precisely the body's... plan B to convert an acidic toxin into a nontoxic alkaline." From the video below: "The term 'chlorine dioxide' is misleading because chlorine is not the active element. Chlorine dioxide is an oxidizing, not a chlorinating agent. ClO_2 penetrates the cell wall and reacts with the amino acids in the cytoplasm within the cell, killing the microorganism. The byproduct of this reaction is chlorite, which is harmless to humans."

Yoho note: I do not understand this either, but there it is.

Cures for AIDS, cancer, Lyme disease, viruses, bacteria, and more have been reported.

The following cannot be dismissed:

❂ In mice and human studies, CD kills certain cancer tumors in less than 48 hours

❂ It kills bacteria, fungi, Giardia, and parasites in humans and animals

✪ Kills viruses, including influenza, Covid, and others

✪ Prevents viral illnesses

✪ Treats infected wounds and improves wound healing time

✪ CD is used as a sanitizing agent and for producing sterile water

✪ Treats HIV, but most countries do not allow this

✪ Treats HPV—genital warts

✪ Kills multi-drug resistant bacteria

✪ Treats pseudomonas, e coli, staph aureus

✪ CD can be used to decontaminate deep surgical wounds and cure surgical infections

✪ Cures toenail fungus and candida. You can order a commercial product HERE.

✪ Cures fungal skin infections. When sprayed on the entire body, all funguses are cured

✪ Treats viral hepatitis

✪ Cures inflammatory diseases such as rheumatoid arthritis

✪ Cures malaria within three hours to three days in 154 out of 154 people in one study. The International Red Cross covered this up. The video documentary about it has been banned from YouTube, but the links to the Bitchute and Brighteon versions can be found below. One provider describes treating 500 people in a day.

✪ Missionaries in Africa report curing 70,000 to 100,000 cases of typhoid fever and malaria

✪ Curing chronic, debilitating Lyme disease

✪ Treats diabetes

✪ Potentially cures inflammatory arthritis

✪ Cures or or nearly cures herpes (Alcide Corporation)

✪ For seriously ill Covid patients, CD rapidly cured 100/100 patients in Ecuador and thousands more without a failure. This was documented in a study.

✪ CD has been reported to restore bladder control in women who have stress incontinence

✪ Cures chronic fatigue

✪ Kalcker says it prevents some of the potential harms from the graphene oxide in the Covid vax

By now, you think I am crazy.

But before you cry BS on my story, watch THIS video from TheUniversalAntidote.com (at double speed, of course). It is the easiest way to understand the backing for chlorine dioxide and its 40-year history. CD works faster and is safer against bacteria and viruses than antibiotics. It has cured Covid for tens of thousands of patients and healed hundreds of thousands with other conditions.

This video shows dozens of testimonials from people who were cured by chlorine dioxide. Anyone who claims these are "simply anecdotes" has adopted the language of the psychopaths. Here is another example. After childhood vaccinations, over 10,000 US children fell to the ground, started banging their heads, and never spoke again. First-hand evidence like this is far better proof than a sack of clinical trials, for two-thirds of federally or Pharma-funded trials are faked.

DOWNLOAD (from ebook) the *Universal Antidote Interactive Reference Guidebook* (2nd edition, 2022). It has links to censored sources.

Kalcker's mentor was Jim Humble, an engineer.

While prospecting for gold in the Guyana jungle, 400 miles from any hospital, two members of Jim's team got malaria. They were delirious and had high fevers, but the group had no medications. Humble had only a drinking water disinfectant, sodium chlorite* ($NaClO_2$). He gave his crew a few drops each, and after four hours, they all recovered from one of the worst infectious diseases known. When Mr. Humble also fell ill, it also worked for him.

He was so impressed that he spent years experimenting on himself and others. He discovered that many conditions and infectious diseases responded. Humble began promoting and selling his discovery as the "Miracle Mineral Solution (MMS)."

Mr. Humble wrote several books and arranged to remove their copyright upon his death. I bought them for you, and you should download them immediately:

MMS Health Recovery Guidebook (2016) Download (ebook)

Master Mineral Solution 3rd Millennium (2011) Download

If you want to pay, use THIS LINK.

By 2019, as he revised his last book, Jim Humble had spent 20 years using, studying, and teaching about CD. When he understood the forces against effective and inexpensive treatments, he started the "Genesis 2 Church of Health and Healing." It was an attempt to shield his organization and ideas using freedom of religion. He said MMS was a sacrament but admitted publicly that his organization had nothing to do with religion.

Humble was a flamboyant character who could be mistaken for a televangelist, and his claims seemed exaggerated or even fraudulent. Federal prosecutors took his organization apart, extradited some of his people from South America, and threw them in prison. The NYT's article was "Family Sentenced for Selling Bleach as a Miracle Covid-19 Cure."

Today, chlorine dioxide users are getting away from Humble's promotional style and his "miracle" terminology. Also, the newer method of making CD dissolved in water popularized by Kalcker makes a compound that produces less stomach irritation. (Both work equally well; however, for some uses, such as autism, the older one may have more potent effects.) Although Humble's methods worked and revealed chlorine dioxide's vast potential, the overriding goal today is towards credibility and more widespread acceptance.

Mr. Humble died in 2023 at 91 after a lifetime of service.

Malign forces stand against chlorine dioxide

Several companies developed uses for chlorine dioxide. Alcide Corporation perfected, patented, and sold many of them, but in 2004, Echolab, a multibillion-dollar company, acquired it. They shut down most human research to focus on agricultural and animal use. We cannot be sure the globalists were behind this, but in the context of the smear campaigns, it smells like it.

CD has the potential to replace a lot of expensive doctors and "healthcare." Pharma companies and their lapdog US government agencies are covering this up. Patent drugs are more profitable, but there is more to the story:

✪ Chlorine dioxide could cure or limit the effects of Lyme, Covid, and the Covid "vaccine." These are bioweapons.

✪ After their first dose of chlorine dioxide, some autistic children speak for the first time in years. This makes it the only effective tool that I know of against the autism caused by childhood vaccines. See my interview with Kerri Rivera HERE for more. Note: Kerri reports that CD must be made using the original Humble process for this to work. In her experience, the *solution* (CDS), chlorine dioxide dissolved in water, is less effective.

✪ Dr. Kalcker says CDS oxidizes the graphene oxide component of the Covid "vaccine." Rivera says oral EDTA (Ethylenediaminetetraacetic acid) and/or zeolite should also be used for metals like this. She recommends the Touchstone zeolite brand, but as I noted earlier, zeolite is controversial.

IV EDTA chelation is reportedly effective for this but has caused patient injuries, including kidney failure, when used to treat mercury overload. It is moderately expensive and a hassle.

✪ Chlorine dioxide inactivates another manmade atrocity, glyphosate.

CD is Kryptonite against Rockefeller "healthcare"

To repeat, it potentially cures Lyme, Covid, cancer, parasites, infections, malaria, heavy metal toxicity, neurological diseases, many inflammatory diseases, and even autism and other forms of vaccine injury. It destroys glyphosate and may help eliminate graphene oxide from the body.

If doctors used CD, they could more effectively treat infections and myriad other inflammatory and neurological diseases. If ordinary people used it, they would need doctors only rarely. I would have been a better physician if I had known about it while practicing. I hope I would have considered quitting cosmetic surgery to spread the word.

But for chlorine dioxide to work, we must beat the censors. Copy and paste this essay on your computer, then download the video, documents, and Humble's books. Put the knowledge in your head and the CD ingredients in your kitchen. I am going to see what it does for my arthritis, Parkinson's, glyphosate, and heavy metals exposures.

As you study CD, remember what Pierre Kory said, "A thousand anecdotes become *data.*" I call it *proof.* "Anecdotal" is used to dismiss what we see with our eyes and persuade us to trust authority and "the science." It is the language of our oppressors, and they have been using this tactic for time immemorial.

Augustine of Hippo wrote, "The truth is like a lion; you don't have to defend it. Let it loose; it will defend itself." People in other countries are using chlorine dioxide more and more, and even here in censorship-land, the news is getting out. The hand of Providence is guiding us.

References

The Epilogue tells how to make chlorine dioxide from cheap materials and how to buy commercial products.

✪ Kacper Postawsky's documentary is about how chlorine dioxide is being used worldwide. This is the second easiest source after the video above.

✪ Andreas Kalcker's websites have thousands of pages. He also runs courses for doctors and others.

- AndreasKalcker.com/en/
- Foundation: alk. foundation/es_MX
- Order Kalcker's books in N. America: cleanhandsnj.com
- Order in Europe/Asia: voedia.com/es/
- The Kalcker Institute - courses: en.kalckerinstitute.com
- International network of doctors: comusav.com/usa/
- Odysee Channel with how to make CDS.*
- Clinical studies using CDS. Most concern Covid.
- How CD was invented. Dr. Kalcker's work with cows
- Dr. Kalcker's CDS protocols
- Dr. Kalcker's patent for CDS to treat acute intoxication (i.e., venoms)
- Christian Elliot's podcast on deconstructingconventional.com
- *According to a Reddit post, Odysee just lost a lawsuit with the feds over allegedly illegally trading in securities. The platform is not shutting down but "will most likely move into the hands of parties who do not support our best interests." Download any of the videos you want to preserve. This is easy.

✪ Humble's main website, jimhumble.co and chlorine dioxide forum, mmsforum.io

✪ PubMed has 1326 references about chlorine dioxide. Most of them are toxicity studies that conclude it is safe.

✪ Stephanie Seneff (MIT)'s critical interview: CDS destroys glyphosate and cures autism

"Legal" disclaimer: This information is not medical advice—use it at your own risk and under supervision.

Epilogue: Rescue Yourself

No one is coming to save any of us. We must research as if our lives depend on it, for they do. We will only survive if we use all our wits, cunning, and thinking flexibility.

See you around the study hall. Warning: I have a bad habit of wasting other students' time during my breaks.

Commercial products are "gateway drugs" to understanding chlorine dioxide

FrontierPharm's mouthwash, nail fungus solution, and Snoot! nasal spray are safe, powerful, and effective. These make chlorine dioxide easy to use and remove the guesswork. HERE is the Rumble link to my interview with Valerie Alliger-Bograd and Michelle Herman, the company founders.

Chlorine dioxide treats inflammatory and infectious diseases effectively, but this information is heavily suppressed. The prohibitions against making claims are akin to the rules chiropractors face. In many states, they are forbidden from saying that they treat or cure. They are only allowed to state that they support good health.

To comply with laws like these, Snoot! Spray is marketed as a "nose cleanser," and the Frontier products are for external use only. The big corporations stand against CD, for it threatens their revenues and possibly—hopefully—even their existence. Val and Michelle have had to listen to their lies about chlorine dioxide being bleach for years.

Chlorine dioxide is an old, well-known compound that cannot be patented and is inexpensive to make. It offers no hope of substantial corporate profits, so there is no incentive to study it in the ways Rockefeller Medicine claims is required for credibility. But no studies are necessary. The thousands of success stories are overwhelming evidence that it works. As you learn more about CD, remember Pierre Kory's saying, "A thousand anecdotes become data."

I am in a multi-decade battle to the death with the nail fungus I caught from my climbing shoes. Once a week, I use a Dremel tool to grind it down and then apply the ointment *du jour*. Nothing has worked. I have been so far unwilling to take oral antifungals for fear they would damage my brain and liver. Fluconazole is fluoridated, for God's sake—it's like taking a statin.

Until recently, I assumed my infestation would outlive me. But Frontier Pharma's product is slowly turning the tide, and I am enjoying poisoning my fellow traveler. (Note: Toenail fungus is often challenging to treat because the problem is systemic.)

I have friends with mouth problems, and they say that Frontier's mouthwash is helping them. Val gets grateful phone calls every week.

Valerie and Michelle are far from rich and nearly abandoned their business in frustration two years ago. Their company faces the same growth problems as any startup—how does it bootstrap and grow? To sell their products, Frontier and Snoot recently started affiliate sales. This incentivizes the small but vocal group who understands CD. Growth rather than short-term profit is the goal.

Some related sales arrangements require an upfront 'investment' then hawk humdrum or nearly useless household products. Chlorine dioxide is different—it potentially has a huge impact on health and is virtually unknown. Frontier Pharm and Snoot require no purchase requirement, minimum order, or "starter package" to join. Here is how it works: when you click my affiliate link below, buy mouthwash, toothpaste, and Snoot! Spray or other product, you get a five percent discount, and I get a commission that I give away to educators who promote chlorine dioxide and other Freedom Movement people.

I signed up and received $2500 in the first several weeks. If you give your commissions away as well, the word might spread more rapidly, and maybe fortune will smile on you. But if this does not appeal to you, please keep your earnings.

Use my links to join the programs:

- My affiliate link HERE takes you to the Frontier website to buy their mouthwash and other products.

- THIS ONE is for the Snoot! Spray nasal products.

- If you want to help spread the word and make money, join the Frontier affiliate program HERE.

- Snoot!'s program is HERE.

After you fill out the application forms to become an affiliate, you will be sent a link to your dashboard in less than a day. There, you will find special website access links to send to your friends or use on your written announcements. These will give you credit for their orders, and your customers will get the introductory discount. You can also make a personal code to use when you podcast or do other speaking.

Legal note for you: If you join the Frontier or the Snoot! Spray group, never say their products treat or cure disease. This is frowned upon by regulators. Val, Michelle, and their companies make no therapeutic claims.

Contacts

Michelle Herman, Snootspray.com; Owner and President. Michelle@snootspray.com

Valerie Alliger-Bograd, Owner and President of Frontier Pharmaceutical, Inc., vab@frontierpharm.com Frontierpharm.com, O: 631-367-3400

Learn to make chlorine dioxide solution (CDS) in your kitchen:

The following videos show a method of dissolving pure CD in water popularized by Andreas Kalcker:

✪ HERE (https://odysee.com/@Truewholehuman:c/Chlorine-Dioxide-Tutorial-2:2--Christian Elliot from Truewholehuman.com)

✪ HERE

✪ HERE

The process happens inside a sealed jar or bottle surrounded by water. The CD gas that is produced saturates the water. The solution can last many months if refrigerated in a sealed brown bottle.

Jim Humble invented a way to make a closely related but stronger preparation, dilute sodium chlorite ($NaClO_2$) solution. Sodium chlorite 22.5 percent is mixed with an "acid activator.*" A minute later, it is ready to dilute and consume. Although this is effective and most people tolerate it well, it has an unpleasant taste and can occasionally cause stomach upset, diarrhea, and, rarely, vomiting. However, according to Kerri Rivera, it is more effective than CDS against autism and possibly other severe conditions. People over 50 should avoid side effects by sticking with CDS.

Humble caused confusion by inventing multiple names for his creation. He called the above "Miracle Mineral Solution (MMS)" and Kalcker's pure CDS "activated MMS." THIS LINK may be more than you need to know about MMS.

*Four percent hydrochloric acid is best, but alternatively, lemon juice, lime juice, or vinegar (5% acetic acid) may be used. Citric acid

50% works but causes more side effects unless you are making a CD solution as above.

See my Substack article HERE for more.

To obtain ingredients:

✪ Buy pre-made CDS solution for "water purification" HERE.

✪ For $200 or less, you can get half gallons of sodium chlorite 22.5% and hydrochloric acid 4% from chemical companies selling on Ebay and elsewhere. You can make enough CDS or CD for your entire neighborhood for years.

✪ A simple manufacturing method using a tablet added to a base solution is HERE.

✪ Amazon sells small amounts of these ingredients in dropper bottles, but many links have been censored. HERE is one that still works.

How Andreas Kalcker's followers fire their dentists

Testimonial from *Forbidden Health* (2018), pages 175-6 (abridged for clarity).

A few months ago, one of my fillings fell out. I didn't go to the dentist for about a week... eating was very painful. By the time I went to the dentist, the pain was unbearable and had extended to my jaw. My dentist removed the remnants of the filling and fixed my tooth with resin, as requested. I wanted to remove all the metal from my mouth...

I went back a week later since I still had pain from eating... My dentist said there was no option except to pull the tooth or do a root canal. I... said, "Give me one week..." I started the following procedure:

Put 1 ml of CDS in a small glass and add 1.5 ounces (45 cc) of distilled water. (If CDS is unavailable, use MMS and wait at least one minute before adding the water.) Add 20 drops of 70% DMSO. If your DMSO is 99% pure, dilute it to 70% by adding 30% distilled water.

Put this solution in your mouth and hold it over the affected tooth for one and a half minutes, then spit it out. You may rinse with distilled water, but this is not necessary. Repeat this procedure at least three times a day, especially after each meal and brushing your teeth.

You may notice an improvement the same day. In about 48 hours, the pain should disappear. Depending on the degree of infection, continue for about five more days. If the tooth bothers you again, continue for two or three more days.

My tooth is safe and sound, and I do not need a root canal.

How Debbie Butler is curing her health problems, conclusion:

I went to a biological dentist, and after an eight-hour struggle, he removed three root canals and a dead tooth that had a mercury filling.

I immediately felt better. All my numbness and other symptoms that began when I had my third root canal placed about two years earlier started to fade. My mummified teeth had been suppressing my immunity, and when the third one was placed, I must have crossed my resistance threshold, and I became sick.

After my teeth were extracted, my nose stopped running, and I stopped sneezing. Dr. Schroeder had the same experience when he had his amalgams removed.

The dentist sent the teeth for a $1000 DNA examination. (Yoho note: Similar tests are available in Europe for about $300 at Armin-labs.com.) It returned positive for three (3) tick-borne species related to Borrelia burgdorferi, the Lyme spirochete. These were Borrelia recurentis, Babesia duncani, and Babesia microti.

Judging by my symptoms, I had been infected for at least 12 years. When I broke my leg in the 2014 auto accident, my toe tingling turned into severe neuropathy. I learned that trauma and even stress can activate tick disease. I must have crossed my resistance threshold again.

A few months after my 2021 accident and a revision knee replacement, I was orthopedically improved but still had pain in my legs and numbness in most of my body, including the inside of my mouth. I could hardly walk. Lyme disease causes neurological problems like this.

I have spent untold hours on Lyme's Facebook pages. One group had 25,000 members. No one seemed to be responding to antibiotics or other Western treatments. Many people were wheelchair- or bed-bound. I quit Facebook because they all seemed hopeless, and I could no longer listen to them.

Then, I stumbled on chlorine dioxide (CD). I saw no success reports on Google despite searching three pages deep. CD seemed like a fraud. But I began reading Dr. Kalcker, who said CD cured Lyme disease. His protocols instructed me to drink chlorine dioxide solution hourly, most of the day, for six weeks or more.

I was desperate, so I tried it. It did smell like bleach. I mixed the 4 percent hydrochloric acid activator and the 25 percent sodium chlorite and drank it all day. Most of my symptoms disappeared on the first day. I had no stomach upset or diarrhea, so I gradually increased my dose. When I returned to Facebook and told my story, they kicked me off.

I consulted with Keri Rivera, a naturopath. She told me to gradually increase my dose to 40 to 80 cc of CDS daily if I tolerated it, diluted in a liter of water. She said it would take many months to cure my problem.

I am at six weeks, and I feel 100 times better. The numbness is slow to improve, but I know nerves take a long time to heal. I am now making chlorine dioxide solution (CDS) using the Kalcker method, and I do not intend to quit.

Once, when Deb missed her CDS for two days, the symptoms came back with a vengeance. She is increasing her dose and hoping that four to six months of treatment will finally cure her.

Note: I am retired, so I give no specific medical advice. This information is for general education only. If you have health problems, find an experienced, licensed provider to treat you. But never check your critical thinking abilities at the door—do your research and participate in your care.

What happened to me?

My colleagues have treated Parkinson's with intravenous stem cells, but the word on the street is that it does not work. My new doctor's approach was to use marrow from the bone below my knee. His team processed the cells and injected them into my arthritic ankles and thirty acupuncture meridians in the front of my body. To reach my brain, the material was dripped in my eyes and squirted deep into my nose.

A week later, my tremor is better and my clumsiness has declined. I am still on intravenous phosphatidylcholine, glutathione, and folinic acid to eliminate heavy metals. Treatments for problems like my wife's and mine require a team effort between the surgeon, dentist, and functional doctors.

First and last: Judy

My life has been filled with adversity, but I hit the jackpot forty years ago when Judy stalked and married me. The Chinese say their women work in the fields all day, then go home to take care of their homes and family. Judy did all that, plus she gave me three wonderful kids and was an equal partner in our medical practice. By the end of each week, I was so exhausted that I could barely play doctor, but Judy still had energy to burn.

Recently, I was certain that Judy was dying. But her health has been transformed, and her new teeth are lovely. If I were a better husband, I would never say I am disappointed she doesn't give me more credit.

Climber Rick Ridgeway wrote, "We have time, but it ain't forever." Judy and I cherish our lives because we understand now that nothing lasts. We face the future with new confidence—we know that if Judy can be saved, there is hope for the rest of us.

We also understand 🤍 better:

When I was a child, I spoke like a child, I thought like a child, I reasoned like a child. When I became a man, I gave up childish ways. For now we see in a mirror dimly, but then face to face. Now I know in part; then I shall know fully, even as I have been fully known.

So now faith, hope, and love abide, these three; but the greatest of these is love.

— 1 Corinthians 13

Please Stay in Touch

I hope we now have a relationship. I am distributing this ebook free HERE at https://dl.bookfunnel.com/5ercuvl94y. If you are not yet using an e-reader, the support people at my service will help you get one. Ebooks are easy and help you find references.

Please write an Amazon review. I will read it, and I appreciate you for doing it. Reviewing a book before finishing is acceptable; you can update later.

Address: 99 West California Blvd #50007, Pasadena, CA 91115, yoho.robert@gmail.com. I will send you more if you subscribe at RobertYoho.substack.com.

Meet the Author

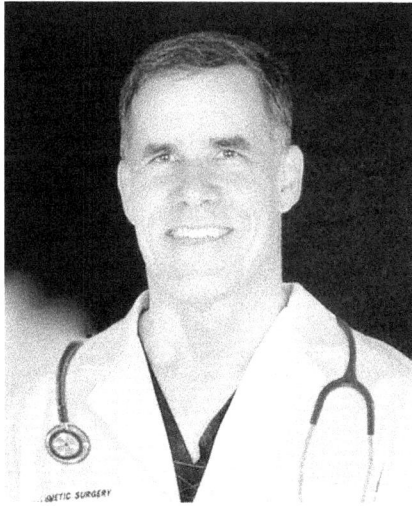

I like my 2010 photo better than today's.

PROFESSIONAL CV:
⭐ Seventy years old (2023). Current website: RobertYohoAuthor.com.

⭐ RobertYoho.substack.com

✪ Emergency medicine career out of medical school.

✪ American Board of Emergency Medicine: passed board exams and twice re-certified.

✪ Practiced three decades as a cosmetic surgeon, now retired (see DrYoho.com).

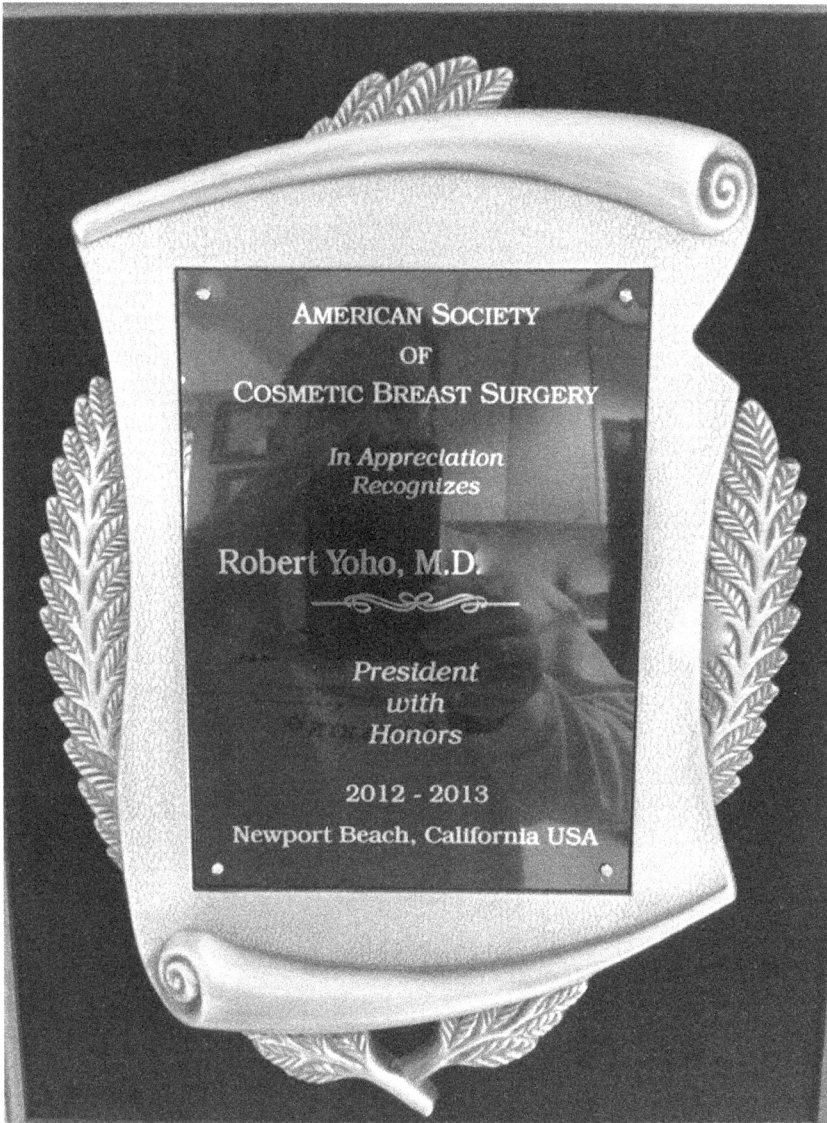

American Society of Cosmetic Breast Surgery: fellow, trustee, officer, and past president.

✪ American Board of Cosmetic Surgery: passed board exams, then twice re-certified.

✪ Fellow, American Academy of Cosmetic Surgery (inactive).

✪ New Body Cosmetic Surgery Center: founder & director (inactive).

✪ American Association of Ambulatory Health Care (AAAHC) accredited surgical/medical practice for over 25 years.

✪ Retired from medical practice in 2019.

* * *

CLIMBER CV:

✪ El Capitan, Half Dome (Yosemite): 24-hour ascents

✪ Free ascents of Astroman (11.c) and Crucifix (12.a)

✪ First ascents in Yosemite, Joshua Tree, Devil's Tower

✪ Solo ascents to 5.10c

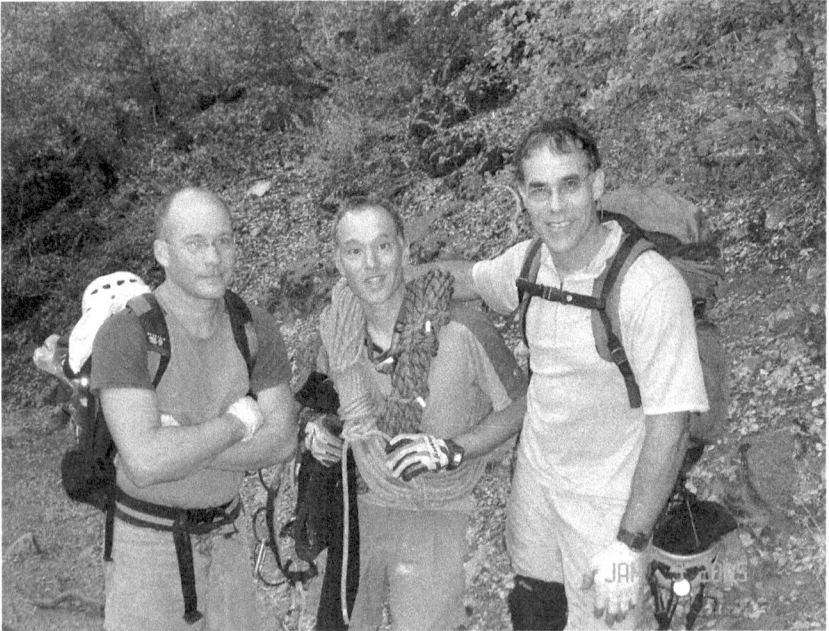

Exhaustion after climbing Yosemite's El Capitan in 26 hours. We are two MDs and a Ph.D.